A COLOUR ATLAS OF
The SKULL

B.K.B. BERKOVITZ
Department of Anatomy
King's College, London

B.J. MOXHAM
Department of Anatomy
University of Bristol

Photography by
D. Telling
Department of Anatomy
University of Bristol

WOLFE MEDICAL PUBLICATIONS LTD

Copyright © B.K.B. Berkovitz, B.J. Moxham, 1989
First published 1989 by Wolfe Medical Publications Ltd
Printed by W.S. Cowell Ltd, Ipswich, England
ISBN 0 7234 0983 8

A CIP catalogue record for this book is available from the British Library.

This book is one of the titles in the series of Wolfe Medical Atlases, a series
that brings together the world's largest systematic published collection of
diagnostic colour photographs.

For a full list of Wolfe Medical Atlases, plus forthcoming titles and details of
our surgical, dental and veterinary Atlases, please write to Wolfe Medical
Publications Ltd, 2-16 Torrington Place, London WC1E 7LT, England.

PREFACE

Human skeletal material is becoming
increasingly difficult to obtain.
This manual provides complete coverage of the
articulated skull, the individual bones of the skull,
and the teeth to help compensate for the
lack of this type of material. The skull is shown
in a series of life-size colour pictures. For the
articulated skull, each view is accompanied by a
full size radiograph. To avoid obscuring
structures, labelling is presented on
accompanying line drawings.

CONTENTS

INTRODUCTION

The skull is the bony skeleton of the head and is the most complex osseous structure in the body. It protects the brain, the organs of special sense and the cranial parts of the respiratory and digestive systems. The skull also provides attachments for many of the muscles of the head and neck.

Although often thought of as a single bone, the skull is composed of 28 separate bones. Many of these are flat bones, consisting of two thin plates of compact bone enclosing a narrow layer of cancellous bone. In terms of shape, however, the bones are far from flat and can show pronounced curvatures. The term diploë is used to describe the cancellous bone within the flat bones of the skull.

In order to make the skull easier to understand, two major subdivisions have been proposed. First, one can subdivide the skull into cranium and mandible. This subdivision is based upon the fact that, whereas most of the bones of the skull articulate by relatively fixed joints, the mandible is easily detached. The cranium may then itself be subdivided into a number of regions, including:

- The cranial vault: The upper, dome-like part of the skull (including the skullcap or calvaria).
- The cranial base: The inferior surface of the skull extracranially, and the floor of the cranial cavity intracranially.
- The facial skeleton: The face (including the orbital cavities and the nasal fossae).
- The jaws: The tooth-bearing bones.
- The acoustic cavities: The ears.
- The cranial cavity: The interior of the skull housing the brain.

Second, one can subdivide the skull into neurocranium and viscerocranium. The neurocranium is defined as that part of the skull that houses and protects the brain and the organs of special sense. The viscerocranium is that region associated with the cranial parts of the respiratory and digestive tracts.

THE NORMA FRONTALIS

Most of the features seen on the front of the skull relate to the face. In particular, there are four apertures associated with the facial skeleton: the two orbital apertures, the anterior nasal aperture (the piriform aperture), and the oral aperture between the jaws.

The upper part of the facial skeleton is formed by the frontal bone and is related to the forehead. Above the bridge of the nose lies a slight elevation called the glabella. This part of the frontal bone joins the nasal bones and the frontal processes of the maxillary bones at the frontonasal and frontomaxillary sutures. At the superior rim of each orbit are found the supra-orbital foramen (or notch) and the frontal notch. These transmit the supra-orbital and supratrochlear nerves (and accompanying vessels) from the orbit on to the forehead. Laterally, the zygomatic processes of the frontal bone join the cheek bones (zygomatic bones) at the frontozygomatic sutures.

The central part of the face is occupied by the maxillary bones. Each bone contributes not only to the upper jaw, but also to the nasal aperture, the bridge of the nose, the floor of an orbital cavity and the bones of the cheek. Beneath the inferior rim of each orbit lies the infra-orbital foramen. Through this foramen, the infra-orbital nerve and accompanying vessels pass on to the face. At the inferior margin of the nasal aperture in the midline lies a projection called the anterior nasal spine. The maxillary bones meet at the intermaxillary suture.

The lower part of the face is formed by the body of the mandible. In the midline is the prominence of the chin, the mental protuberance. In line with the supra-orbital and infra-orbital foramina lies the mental foramen. Through this foramen passes the mental nerve (and accompanying vessels).

The muscles attached to the front of the skull are:

MUSCLE	ATTACHED TO:
BUCCINATOR	Maxillary and mandibular buccal alveolar plates in region of molars
CORRUGATOR SUPERCILII	Frontal bone
DEPRESSOR ANGULI ORIS	Mandible below mental foramen
DEPRESSOR LABII INFERIORIS	Mandible between chin and mental foramen
DEPRESSOR SEPTI	Maxilla below nasal aperture
LEVATOR ANGULI ORIS	Maxilla below infra-orbital foramen
LEVATOR LABII SUPERIORIS	Inferior rim of orbit above infra-orbital foramen
LEVATOR LABII SUPERIORIS ALAEQUE NASI	Frontal process of maxilla
MASSETER	Zygomatic arch and lateral surface of ramus of mandible
MENTALIS	Incisive fossa of mandible
NASALIS	Maxilla close to nasal aperture
ORBICULARIS OCULI	Nasal part of the frontal bone, frontal process of maxilla and crest of lacrimal bone
PLATYSMA	Inferior border of body of mandible
PROCERUS	Nasal bone
TEMPORALIS	Temporal fossa and coronoid process and anterior border of ramus
ZYGOMATICUS MAJOR	Zygomatic bone
ZYGOMATICUS MINOR	Zygomatic bone

NORMA FRONTALIS

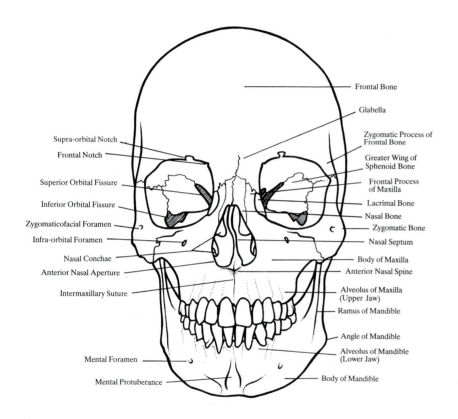

- Frontal Bone
- Glabella
- Zygomatic Process of Frontal Bone
- Greater Wing of Sphenoid Bone
- Frontal Process of Maxilla
- Lacrimal Bone
- Nasal Bone
- Zygomatic Bone
- Nasal Septum
- Body of Maxilla
- Anterior Nasal Spine
- Alveolus of Maxilla (Upper Jaw)
- Ramus of Mandible
- Angle of Mandible
- Alveolus of Mandible (Lower Jaw)
- Body of Mandible

- Supra-orbital Notch
- Frontal Notch
- Superior Orbital Fissure
- Inferior Orbital Fissure
- Zygomaticofacial Foramen
- Infra-orbital Foramen
- Nasal Conchae
- Anterior Nasal Aperture
- Intermaxillary Suture
- Mental Foramen
- Mental Protuberance

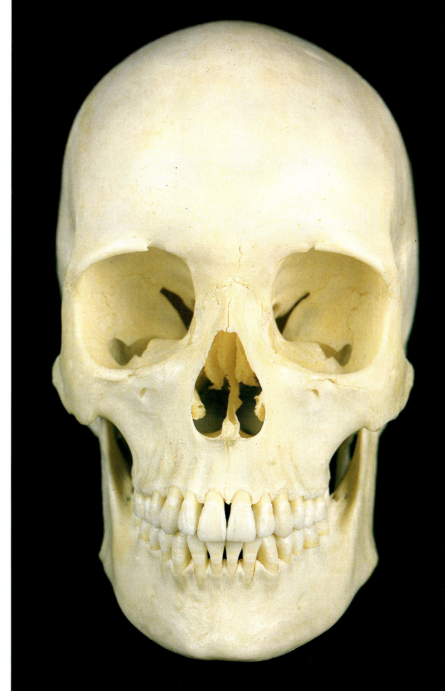

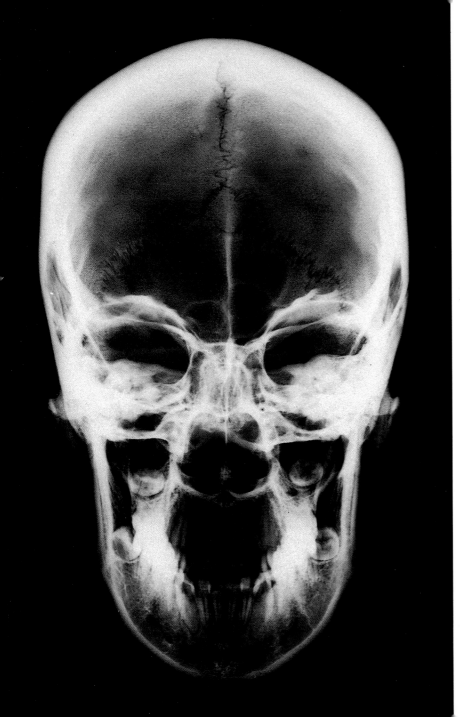

POSTEROANTERIOR RADIOGRAPH OF SKULL

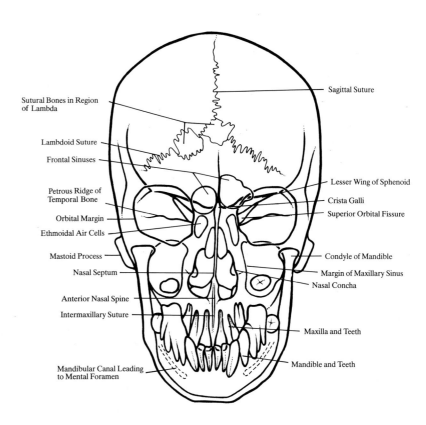

Sutural Bones in Region of Lambda

Lambdoid Suture

Frontal Sinuses

Petrous Ridge of Temporal Bone

Orbital Margin

Ethmoidal Air Cells

Mastoid Process

Nasal Septum

Anterior Nasal Spine

Intermaxillary Suture

Mandibular Canal Leading to Mental Foramen

Sagittal Suture

Lesser Wing of Sphenoid

Crista Galli

Superior Orbital Fissure

Condyle of Mandible

Margin of Maxillary Sinus

Nasal Concha

Maxilla and Teeth

Mandible and Teeth

THE NORMA LATERALIS

The skull, viewed from the side, can be subdivided into three zones. Anteriorly is the face, and posteriorly is the occipital region. The intermediate zone shows two fossae: the temporal and infratemporal fossae. The boundary between the fossae is the zygomatic arch.

The upper part of the skull (or calvaria) is comprised of the frontal bone, two parietal bones and the occipital bone. The frontal bone meets the parietal bones at the coronal suture. The occipital bone meets the parietal bones at the lambdoid suture. The calvaria is described later with the norma verticalis (page 33).

The temporal fossa is so named because it is related to the temple of the head. The fossa is bounded inferiorly by the zygomatic arch; superiorly and posteriorly by the temporal lines on the calvaria; and anteriorly by the frontal process of the zygomatic bone. It continues beneath the zygomatic arch into the infratemporal fossa. The temporal lines often present anteriorly as distinct ridges but become much less prominent as they arch across the parietal bone. Indeed, the superior line usually disappears posteriorly. On the other hand, the inferior temporal line becomes distinct once more as it curves down the squamous part of the temporal bone,

forming a supramastoid crest at the base of the mastoid process. The superior temporal line gives attachment to the temporal fascia. The inferior temporal line provides attachment for the temporalis muscle.

The floor of the temporal fossa is formed by the frontal, sphenoid (greater wing), parietal and temporal (squamous part) bones. These four bones meet at an area called the pterion, where there is an H-shaped junction of sutures. This is an important landmark on the side of the skull. It overlies the middle meningeal vessels intracranially and corresponds to the sphenoidal fontanelle on the neonatal skull.

The suture between the temporal and parietal bones is called the squamosal suture. The sphenosquamosal suture lies between the greater wing of the sphenoid and the squamous part of the temporal bone.

The infratemporal fossa has the following bony boundaries: the ramus of the mandible laterally; the lateral pterygoid plate of the sphenoid bone medially; the infratemporal surface of the greater wing of the sphenoid superiorly; and the maxilla anteriorly. Beneath the zygomatic arch, the infratemporal fossa communicates with the temporal fossa. Between the lateral pterygoid plate and the maxilla lies the pterygomaxillary fissure. This fissure marks the site where the infratemporal fossa communicates with the pterygopalatine fossa.

The ramus of the mandible is a plate of bone projecting upwards from the back of the body of the mandible. Most of its lateral surface provides attachment for the masseter muscle. Two prominent processes are seen superiorly, the coronoid and condylar processes. The coronoid process is the site for the insertion of the temporalis muscle. The condylar process articulates with the mandibular fossa of the temporal bone at the temporomandibular synovial joint. Between the two processes is the mandibular notch. The angle of the mandible is the region where the inferior and posterior borders of the ramus meet.

The zygomatic arch stands clear of the rest of the skull, the gap being where the temporal and infratemporal fossae communicate. Whereas the bones of the cheek comprise the zygomatic bone and the zygomatic processes of the frontal, maxillary and temporal bones, the zygomatic arch is a term restricted to that part formed by the temporal process of the zygomatic bone and the zygomatic process of the temporal bone. These processes meet at the zygomaticotemporal suture. The suture between the frontal process of the zygomatic bone and the zygomatic process of the frontal bone is called the frontozygomatic suture. The zygomaticomaxillary suture marks the union of the maxillary margin of the zygomatic bone and zygomatic process of the maxillary bone. The zygomatic bone also joins the sphenoid bone, at the sphenozygomatic suture. As the zygomatic process of the temporal bone passes posteriorly, it becomes associated with the mandibular fossa and the supramastoid crest.

The upper border of the zygomatic arch serves as an attachment for the temporal fascia. The inferior border and the deep surface provide attachment for the masseter muscle. A small foramen, the zygomaticofacial foramen, lies on the outer surface of the zygomatic bone. Another foramen, the zygomaticotemporal foramen, is situated on the inner surface. These foramina transmit nerves and vessels of the same name on to the face.

The temporal bone is a prominent structure on the lateral aspect of the skull. As mentioned, its squamous part lies in the floor of the temporal fossa and its zygomatic process contributes to the bones of the cheek. Additional features found are the mandibular fossa and its articular tubercle, the tympanic plate and external acoustic meatus, and the mastoid and styloid processes.

The mandibular fossa has also been called the glenoid fossa. It is the part of the temporomandibular joint into which the condylar process of the mandible articulates. It is bounded in front by the articular tubercle and behind by the tympanic plate. Occasionally, there is a postglenoid tubercle. The articular tubercle is important functionally as it provides a surface down which the mandibular condyle glides during mandibular movements. The tubercle also marks the site of attachment of the lateral ligament of the temporomandibular joint.

The tympanic part of the temporal bone contributes most of the margin of the external acoustic meatus, the squamous part forming the upper margin and the upper part of the posterior margin. The margin is roughened to provide an attachment for the cartilaginous part of the meatus. Above and behind the meatus lies a small depression, the suprameatal triangle, which is related to the lateral wall of the mastoid antrum.

The mastoid process is the large prominence located immediately behind the external acoustic meatus. It is the site of attachment of a prominent muscle of the neck, the sternocleidomastoid muscle. Above the process lies the supramastoid crest. The mastoid process articulates with the parietal and occipital bones at the parietomastoid and occipitomastoid sutures. The junction of these sutures with the lambdoid suture is called the asterion. This corresponds to the mastoid fontanelle in the neonatal skull. A mastoid foramen may be found near the occipitomastoid suture. This foramen transmits an emissary vein from the sigmoid sinus.

The styloid process is a long, slender process that emerges from the base of the skull in front of the mastoid process. It projects downwards and forwards towards the mandible. The base of the styloid process is formed by the tympanic part of the temporal bone. The process gives attachment to several muscles and ligaments.

The muscles attached to the lateral side of the skull are:

MUSCLE	ATTACHED TO:
BUCCINATOR	Maxillary and mandibular buccal alveolar plates in region of molars
CORRUGATOR SUPERCILII	Frontal bone
DEPRESSOR ANGULI ORIS	Mandible below mental foramen
DEPRESSOR LABII INFERIORIS	Mandible between chin and mental foramen
DEPRESSOR SEPTI	Maxilla below nasal aperture
LEVATOR ANGULI ORIS	Maxilla below the infra-orbital foramen
LEVATOR LABII SUPERIORIS	Inferior rim of orbit above infra-orbital foramen
LEVATOR LABII SUPERIORIS ALAEQUE NASI	Frontal process of maxilla
MASSETER	Zygomatic arch, lateral surface of mandibular ramus
MENTALIS	Incisive fossa of mandible
NASALIS	Maxilla close to nasal aperture
OCCIPITAL BELLY OF. OCCIPITOFRONTALIS	Superior nuchal line
ORBICULARIS OCULI	Nasal part of frontal bone, frontal process of maxilla and crest of lacrimal bone
PLATYSMA	Inferior border of body of mandible
PROCERUS	Nasal bone
STERNOCLEIDOMASTOID	Mastoid process, superior nuchal line
TEMPORALIS	Temporal fossa, coronoid process of mandible and anterior border of ramus
ZYGOMATICUS MAJOR	Zygomatic bone
ZYGOMATICUS MINOR	Zygomatic bone

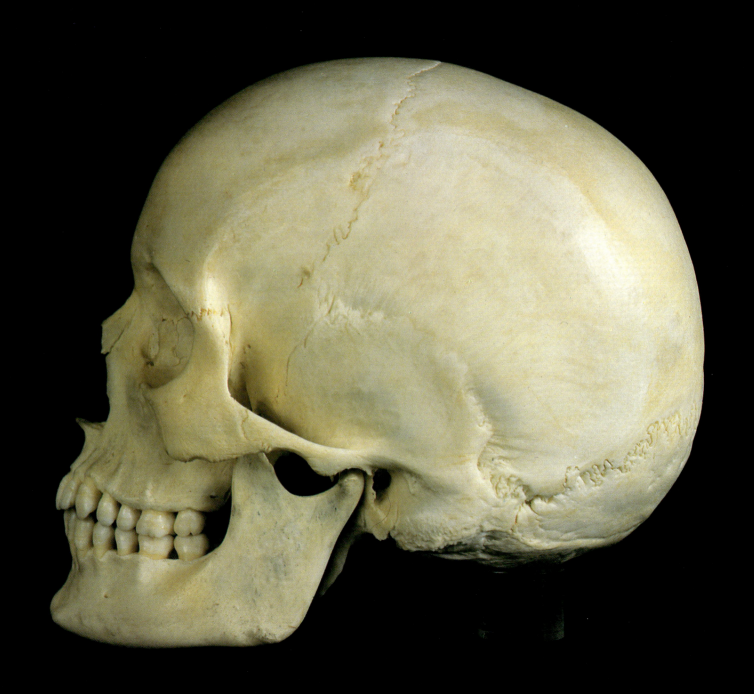

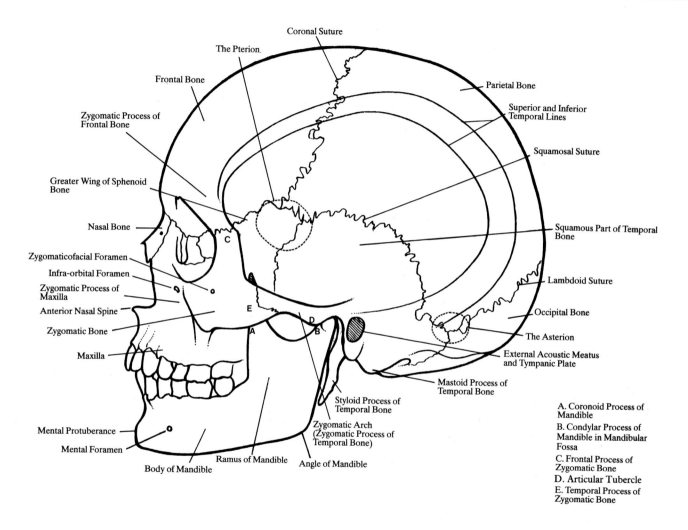

Coronal Suture

The Pterion

Frontal Bone

Parietal Bone

Superior and Inferior
Temporal Lines

Zygomatic Process of
Frontal Bone

Squamosal Suture

Greater Wing of Sphenoid
Bone

Nasal Bone

Squamous Part of Temporal
Bone

Zygomaticofacial Foramen

Infra-orbital Foramen

Zygomatic Process of
Maxilla

Anterior Nasal Spine

Zygomatic Bone

Lambdoid Suture

Occipital Bone

The Asterion

Maxilla

External Acoustic Meatus
and Tympanic Plate

Mental Protuberance

Mastoid Process of
Temporal Bone

Mental Foramen

Styloid Process of
Temporal Bone

Zygomatic Arch
(Zygomatic Process of
Temporal Bone)

Body of Mandible

Ramus of Mandible

Angle of Mandible

A. Coronoid Process of
Mandible

B. Condylar Process of
Mandible in Mandibular
Fossa

C. Frontal Process of
Zygomatic Bone

D. Articular Tubercle

E. Temporal Process of
Zygomatic Bone

15

LATERAL RADIOGRAPH OF SKULL

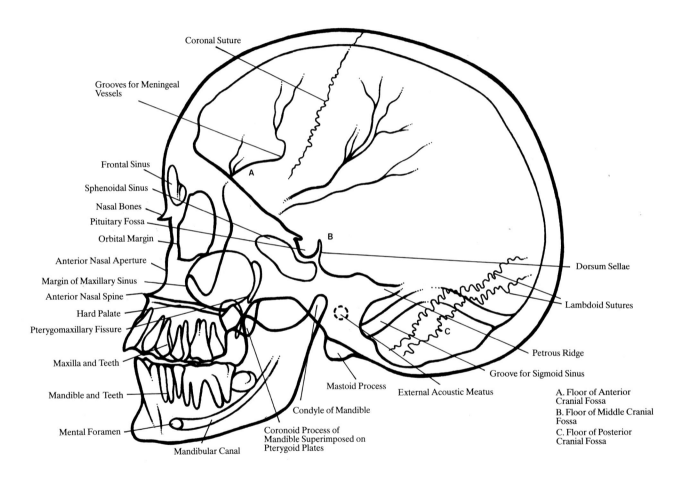

Coronal Suture

Grooves for Meningeal Vessels

Frontal Sinus

Sphenoidal Sinus

Nasal Bones

Pituitary Fossa

Orbital Margin

Anterior Nasal Aperture

Margin of Maxillary Sinus

Anterior Nasal Spine

Hard Palate

Pterygomaxillary Fissure

Maxilla and Teeth

Mandible and Teeth

Mental Foramen

Mandibular Canal

Coronoid Process of Mandible Superimposed on Pterygoid Plates

Condyle of Mandible

Mastoid Process

External Acoustic Meatus

Groove for Sigmoid Sinus

Petrous Ridge

Lambdoid Sutures

Dorsum Sellae

A. Floor of Anterior Cranial Fossa

B. Floor of Middle Cranial Fossa

C. Floor of Posterior Cranial Fossa

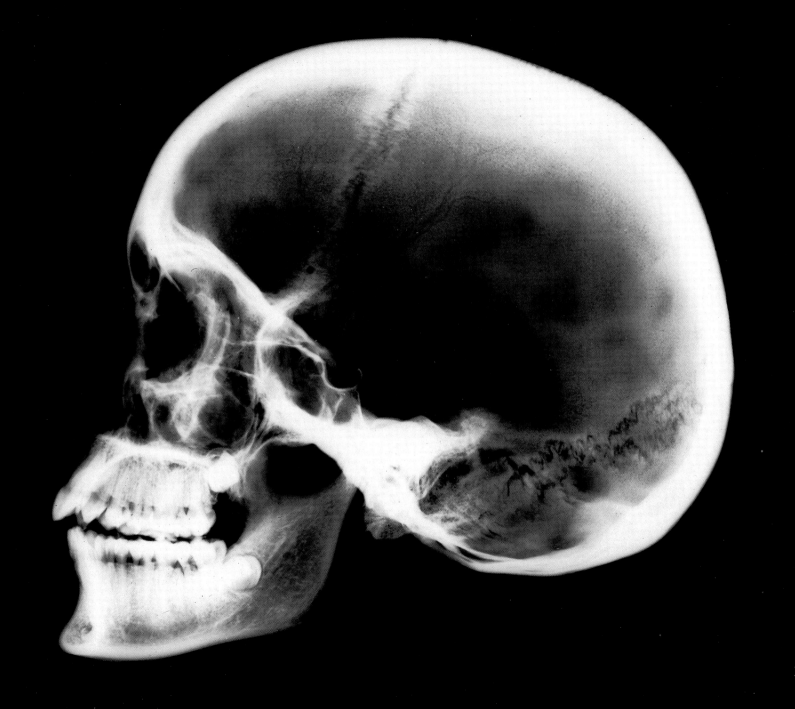

THE NORMA OCCIPITALIS

When the skull is viewed from behind, the occipital bone is prominent—hence the term norma occipitalis. The lambdoid suture between the occipital bone and the parietal bones is also conspicuous, being seen in its entirety. A common variation is the presence of islands of bone within the suture. These sutural bones arise from separate centres of ossification, but they have no clinical significance.

The point of meeting of the lambdoid suture and the sagittal suture of the calvaria is termed the lambda. This site marks the position of the posterior fontanelle on the fetal skull.

Inferiorly, the lambdoid suture meets the occipitomastoid and the parietomastoid sutures. These sutures lie above and behind the mastoid process of the temporal bone. The temporal bones, though most clearly seen on the lateral views of the skull, just appear as the mastoid processes to form the inferolateral parts of the back of the skull. The superolateral parts are formed by the parietal bones.

A marked feature at the back of the skull is the external occipital protuberance. It appears on the occipital bone in the midline as either a ridge or a distinct process. Extending laterally from the protuberance are two ridges called the superior nuchal lines. These lines finish above the mastoid processes. Inferior nuchal lines run parallel to, and below, the superior nuchal lines. Above the superior nuchal lines may be seen the supreme nuchal lines. The external occipital protuberance and the nuchal lines are associated with muscle attachments. The supreme nuchal lines afford attachment to the epicranial aponeurosis of the scalp. The roughened appearance of the occipital bone between the nuchal lines is also caused by muscle attachments.

The muscles attached to the skull in the occipital region are:

MUSCLE	ATTACHED TO:
LONGISSIMUS CAPITIS	Superior nuchal line
OBLIQUUS CAPITIS SUPERIOR	Between superior and inferior nuchal lines
OCCIPITAL BELLY OF OCCIPITOFRONTALIS	Superior nuchal line
SEMISPINALIS CAPITIS	Between superior and inferior nuchal lines
SPLENIUS CAPITIS	Superior nuchal line
STERNOCLEIDOMASTOID	Mastoid process and superior nuchal line
TRAPEZIUS	External occipital protuberance and superior nuchal line

NORMA OCCIPITALIS

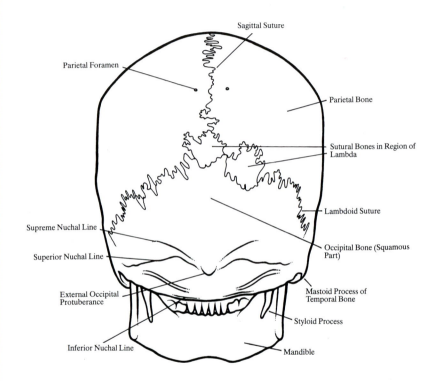

Sagittal Suture

Parietal Foramen

Parietal Bone

Sutural Bones in Region of Lambda

Lambdoid Suture

Supreme Nuchal Line

Superior Nuchal Line

Occipital Bone (Squamous Part)

External Occipital Protuberance

Mastoid Process of Temporal Bone

Styloid Process

Inferior Nuchal Line

Mandible

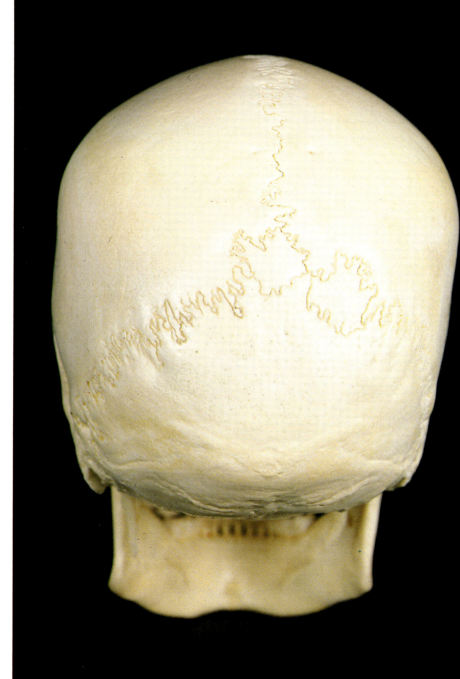

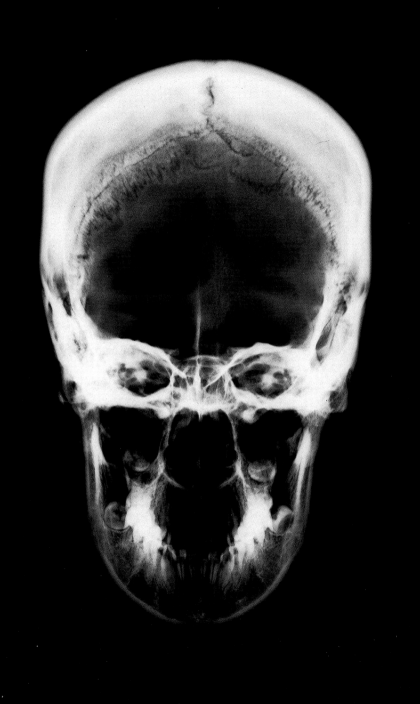

ANTEROPOSTERIOR RADIOGRAPH OF SKULL

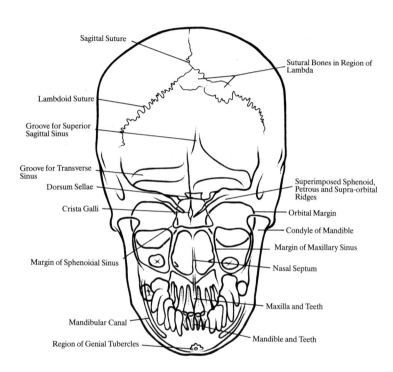

Sagittal Suture

Sutural Bones in Region of Lambda

Lambdoid Suture

Groove for Superior Sagittal Sinus

Groove for Transverse Sinus

Dorsum Sellae

Superimposed Sphenoid, Petrous and Supra-orbital Ridges

Crista Galli

Orbital Margin

Condyle of Mandible

Margin of Maxillary Sinus

Margin of Sphenoidal Sinus

Nasal Septum

Maxilla and Teeth

Mandibular Canal

Region of Genial Tubercles

Mandible and Teeth

THE NORMA BASALIS

The inferior surface of the cranium is very irregular and presents the most complex of the surfaces of the skull. The region can be simplified by subdividing it into three zones. The anterior zone is comprised of the hard palate and the dentition of the upper jaw. The posterior zone lies behind a transverse plane drawn just in front of the foramen magnum. The intermediate zone is occupied mainly by the base of the sphenoid bone, the petrous processes of the temporal bones and the basilar part of the occipital bone. Whereas the intermediate and posterior zones are directly related to the cranial cavity (the middle and posterior cranial fossae), the anterior zone is related to the roof of the mouth and is some distance from the anterior cranial fossa.

The hard palate is formed by the two palatine processes of the maxillary bones and the two horizontal plates of the palatine bones. It is bounded anteriorly and laterally by the alveolus of the upper jaw, which supports the teeth. A cross-shaped set of sutures traverses the palate. Running anteroposteriorly and dividing the palate into right and left halves is the median palatine suture. This suture is continuous with the intermaxillary suture between the maxillary central incisor teeth. Behind the central incisors, the junction between the palatine processes of the maxillary

bones is incomplete, thus forming the incisive fossa. Incisive foramina pass into this fossa and transmit the nasopalatine nerves and the terminal parts of the greater palatine vessels. Running transversely across the palate between the maxillary and the palatine bones is the transverse palatine suture. This suture is incomplete on each side and forms the greater palatine foramina. Through the greater palatine foramen pass the greater palatine nerve and vessels. Behind the foramen lie one or more lesser palatine foramina, through which pass the lesser palatine nerves and vessels. The posterior borders of the horizontal plates of the palatine bones are concave and in the midline form a sharp ridge of bone, the posterior nasal spine.

Above the hard palate are the nasal fossae, separated in the midline by the nasal septum. The posterior part of the septum is formed by the vomer. This bone lies on the body of the sphenoid. Where the nasal fossae end are located the two posterior nasal apertures (choanae). The lateral wall of each aperture beneath the hard palate is formed by the perpendicular plate of the palatine bone. A small canal called the palatovaginal canal is found in this region. This transmits the pharyngeal branch of the pterygopalatine ganglion and an accompanying branch from the maxillary artery. Another canal, the vomerovaginal canal, may sometimes be found leading into the anterior end of the palatovaginal canal. It transmits the pharyngeal branch of the sphenopalatine artery.

A prominent feature of the posterior zone of the cranial base is the foramen magnum. Associated with this foramen are the occipital condyles, the hypoglossal canals (anterior condylar canals) and the condylar canals (posterior condylar canals). Lateral to the foramen magnum are the jugular foramina. Other features of this part of the skull are the mastoid and styloid processes of the temporal bones, the stylomastoid foramina, the mastoid notches and the squamous part of the occipital bone up to the external occipital protuberance and the superior nuchal lines.

The foramen magnum is the largest foramen of the skull. Through it the cranial cavity (the posterior cranial fossa) and the vertebral canal communicate. The major structures passing through the foramen are the medulla oblongata of the brainstem, the vertebral arteries and the spinal accessory nerves.

The occipital condyles lie near the anterior margin of the foramen magnum. They are facets for articulation with the vertebral column at the atlanto-occipital joints. Within each condyle is the hypoglossal canal. This communicates with the posterior cranial fossa and transmits the hypoglossal nerve. It also transmits the meningeal branch of the ascending pharyngeal artery and an emissary vein. Behind each condyle is a depression called the condylar fossa. The condylar canal passes into this fossa and transmits an emissary vein from the sigmoid sinus.

The jugular foramen is an irregular foramen situated lateral to the occipital condyle. Anteriorly, the inferior petrosal sinus passes through the foramen. Midway, the foramen transmits the glossopharyngeal, vagus and accessory nerves. Posteriorly lies the internal jugular vein.

Between the mastoid process and the root of the styloid process is the stylomastoid foramen. Through this foramen emerges the facial nerve. Also passing through is the stylomastoid branch of the posterior auricular artery. Medial to the mastoid process is the mastoid notch. This is the site of attachment of the posterior belly of the digastric muscle. Medial to the notch is a groove in which runs the occipital artery.

The region of the occipital bone between the foramen magnum and the inferior nuchal line provides attachment for the rectus capitis posterior major and minor muscles. Between the inferior and superior nuchal lines are attached the semispinalis capitis and the obliquus capitis superior muscles. The superior nuchal line is the site of attachment of the trapezius, sternocleidomastoid and splenius capitis muscles.

The intermediate zone of the cranial base is essentially comprised of four osseous structures. Anteriorly lies the body of the sphenoid bone, and posteriorly the basilar part of the occipital bone. Where these meet is a primary cartilaginous joint called the spheno-occipital synchondrosis. This joint ossifies at about 20 years of age. The intermediate zone is completed by the petrous processes of the two temporal bones. A petrous process meets the basilar part of the occipital bone at the petro-occipital suture. This suture is deficient posteriorly where the jugular foramen is situated. Between the petrous process and the infratemporal surface of the greater wing of the sphenoid is the sphenopetrosal synchondrosis and the groove for the auditory tube. The apex of the petrous process does not meet the spheno-occipital joint. Consequently, a large fissure is present called the foramen lacerum. The intermediate zone is related to the middle cranial fossa and the anterior wall of the posterior cranial fossa.

The intermediate zone displays a considerable number of fissures and foramina. The foramen lacerum, despite its size, does not transmit any large structures. Its upper part is related to the internal opening of the carotid canal. Thus, the internal carotid artery crosses over the foramen lacerum on its intracranial aspect. The lower part of the foramen lacerum is filled with cartilage. Within the foramen, the greater petrosal branch of the facial nerve and the deep petrosal nerve from the carotid sympathetic plexus join to form the nerve of the pterygoid canal. Indeed, the pterygoid canal can be seen on the base of the skull at the anterior margin of the foramen lacerum, above and between the pterygoid plates of the sphenoid bone. The pterygoid canal leads into the pterygopalatine fossa.

Lateral to the foramen lacerum and passing through the infratemporal surface of the greater wing of the sphenoid are the foramen ovale and the foramen spinosum. The foramen ovale communicates with the middle cranial fossa and contains the mandibular nerve (and also the accessory meningeal artery from the maxillary artery and the lesser petrosal nerve). The foramen spinosum lies anterior to the spine of the sphenoid and posterior to the foramen ovale. It also communicates with the middle cranial fossa. It transmits the middle meningeal vessels and the meningeal branch of the mandibular nerve (nervus spinosus).

Anterior to the foramen ovale a small foramen is sometimes found called the sphenoidal emissary foramen (of Vesalius). This contains an emissary vein linking the pterygoid venous plexus in the infratemporal fossa with the cavernous sinus in the middle cranial fossa.

Behind the foramen lacerum and within the petrous part of the temporal bone is the carotid canal, through which passes the internal carotid artery.

Other features of the intermediate zone are: the pterygoid plates, pterygoid hamulus and scaphoid fossa; the mandibular fossa and its articular tubercle; the petrosquamous, petrotympanic and squamotympanic fissures; the spine of the sphenoid; and the pharyngeal tubercle on the basilar part of the occipital bone.

The pterygoid plates are processes of the sphenoid bone. There are two plates, the lateral and the medial pterygoid plates. They are important for the attachment of muscles. The space between the plates is called the pterygoid fossa. At its base is a depression called the scaphoid fossa, for the attachment of the tensor veli palatini muscle. Anteriorly, the two plates are fused, except for a narrow gap (the pterygoid notch) which is filled by the pyramidal process of the palatine bone. The medial pterygoid plate has a hook-shaped process called the pterygoid hamulus. The tensor veli palatini muscle twists around the hamulus before inserting into the soft palate.

The mandibular fossa appears as a thin-walled depression and the articular tubercle is seen as a distinct ridge anterior to the fossa. Three fissures may be distinguished behind the mandibular fossa. The squamotympanic fissure extends from the spine of the sphenoid, between the mandibular fossa and the tympanic plate of the temporal bone, and up the anterior margin of the external acoustic meatus. Within this fissure may be seen a thin wedge of bone, which is the inferior margin of the tegmen tympani (part of the petrous part of the temporal bone). This divides the squamotympanic fissure into two: the petrotympanic and petrosquamous fissures. The petrotympanic fissure transmits the chorda tympani branch of the facial nerve into the infratemporal fossa.

The spine of the sphenoid is located medial to the mandibular fossa and posterior to the foramen spinosum. It is the site of attachment of the sphenomandibular ligament.

The pharyngeal tubercle is found centrally on the basilar part of the occipital bone. It marks the site of attachment of the highest fibres of the superior constrictor muscle of the pharynx and of the pharyngeal raphe.

The muscles attached to the base of the cranium extracranially are:

MUSCLE	ATTACHED TO:
DIGASTRIC	Mastoid notch
LATERAL PTERYGOID	Lateral side of lateral pterygoid plate and infratemporal surface of greater wing of sphenoid
LEVATOR VELI PALATINI	Petrous part of temporal bone
LONGISSIMUS CAPITIS	Superior nuchal line
LONGUS CAPITIS	Basilar part of occipital bone
MEDIAL PTERYGOID	Medial side of lateral pterygoid plate, tuberosity of maxilla
MUSCULUS UVULAE	Posterior margin of hard palate in midline
OBLIQUUS CAPITIS SUPERIOR	Between superior and inferior nuchal lines
OCCIPITAL BELLY OF OCCIPITOFRONTALIS	Superior nuchal line
PALATOPHARYNGEUS	Posterior margin of hard palate laterally
RECTUS CAPITIS ANTERIOR	Basilar part of occipital bone
RECTUS CAPITIS LATERALIS	Jugular process of occipital bone
RECTUS CAPITIS POSTERIOR MAJOR AND MINOR	Below inferior nuchal line
SEMISPINALIS CAPITIS	Between superior and inferior nuchal lines
SPLENIUS CAPITIS	Superior nuchal line
STERNOCLEIDOMASTOID	Mastoid process, superior nuchal line
STYLOGLOSSUS	Styloid process
STYLOHYOID	Styloid process
STYLOPHARYNGEUS	Styloid process
SUPERIOR CONSTRICTOR	Medial pterygoid plate and pharyngeal tubercle
TENSOR VELI PALATINI	Scaphoid fossa, spine of sphenoid
TRAPEZIUS	External occipital protuberance, superior nuchal line

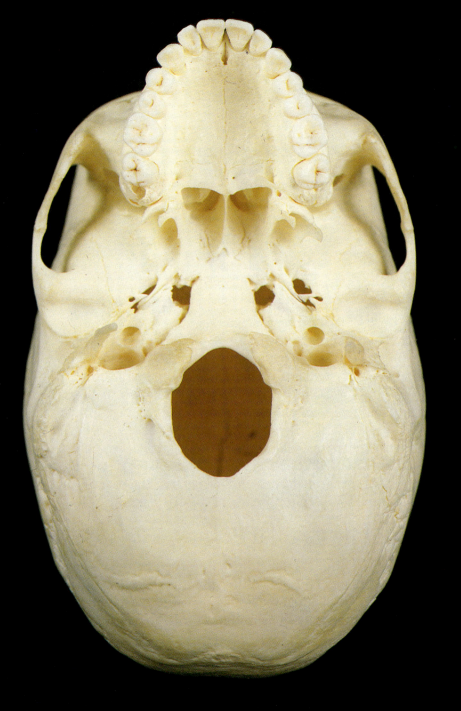

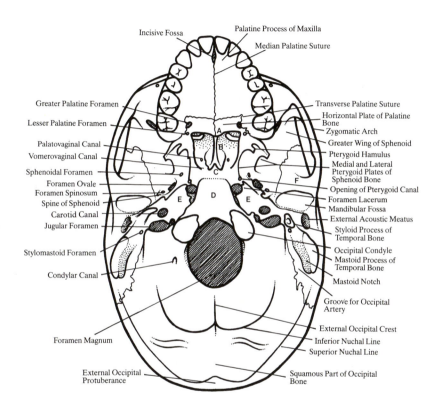

Incisive Fossa

Palatine Process of Maxilla

Median Palatine Suture

Greater Palatine Foramen

Lesser Palatine Foramen

Palatovaginal Canal

Vomerovaginal Canal

Sphenoidal Foramen

Foramen Ovale

Foramen Spinosum

Spine of Sphenoid

Carotid Canal

Jugular Foramen

Stylomastoid Foramen

Condylar Canal

Foramen Magnum

External Occipital Protuberance

Transverse Palatine Suture

Horizontal Plate of Palatine Bone

Zygomatic Arch

Greater Wing of Sphenoid

Pterygoid Hamulus

Medial and Lateral Pterygoid Plates of Sphenoid Bone

Opening of Pterygoid Canal

Foramen Lacerum

Mandibular Fossa

External Acoustic Meatus

Styloid Process of Temporal Bone

Occipital Condyle

Mastoid Process of Temporal Bone

Mastoid Notch

Groove for Occipital Artery

External Occipital Crest

Inferior Nuchal Line

Superior Nuchal Line

Squamous Part of Occipital Bone

A. Posterior Nasal Spine

B. Vomer contributing to Nasal Septum

C. Body of Sphenoid

D. Basilar Part of Occipital Bone

E. Petrous Processes of Temporal Bones

F. Articular Tubercle

THE INTRACRANIAL APPEARANCE OF THE SKULL

The cranial cavity of the skull accommodates the brain and associated structures. It can be divided into anterior, middle and posterior cranial fossae. The three fossae have a marked step-like appearance, such that the floor of the anterior cranial fossa is at the highest level and the floor of the posterior fossa is lowest.

The Anterior Cranial Fossa

The floor of the anterior cranial fossa is formed by the frontal bone (orbital part), the ethmoid bone (cribriform plates and crista galli) and the sphenoid bone (lesser wings and jugum). Unlike the other cranial fossae, it does not directly communicate with the inferior surface of the cranium but instead is related to the roofs of the orbits and the nasal fossae. Two sutures divide the sphenoid from the other bones: the frontosphenoid suture and the spheno-ethmoidal suture. The cribriform plate of the ethmoid bone fills a gap (the ethmoidal notch) between the medial ends of the orbital parts of the frontal bone and is depressed below the level of the rest of the floor. Extending upwards from the cribriform plate is a process called the crista galli. This serves as a point of attachment of the falx cerebri.

There are two openings in the floor of the anterior cranial fossa: the cribriform plates and the foramen caecum. The cribriform plates transmit olfactory nerves into the roof of the nose. The foramen caecum lies immediately in front of the crista galli. It occasionally allows the passage of an emissary vein linking the superior sagittal venous sinus to the veins in the nose. The anterior ethmoidal nerve enters the cranial cavity where the cribriform plate meets the orbital part of the frontal bone and passes into the roof of the nose by a small foramen to the side of the crista galli.

The Middle Cranial Fossa

The floor of the middle cranial fossa is formed by the body of the sphenoid bone centrally and by the greater wings of the sphenoid and the squamous and petrous parts of the temporal bones laterally. The middle cranial fossa is directly related extracranially to the intermediate zone of the cranial base.

In the midline, the prominent structure is the pituitary fossa (sella turcica). This fossa is situated in the upper surface of the body of the sphenoid bone. The anterior slope of the pituitary fossa has an elevation called the tuberculum sellae. In front of the tuberculum sellae is the prechiasmatic groove, which is associated with the optic chiasma and which leads into the optic canals. The pituitary fossa is bounded posteriorly by a plate of bone called the dorsum sellae. Lateral to the pituitary fossa is a groove (the carotid groove) for the internal carotid artery. Anterior and posterior clinoid processes occupy the 'four corners' of the pituitary fossa. These provide sites of attachment for a sheet of the meninges called the diaphragma sellae, which roofs over the pituitary fossa.

The regions lateral to the pituitary fossa provide deep depressions for the temporal lobes of the brain. Each region is related to the apex of the orbit anteriorly, the temporal fossa laterally and the infratemporal fossa inferiorly.

The openings of the middle cranial fossa on each side are: the optic canal, superior orbital fissure, foramen rotundum, foramen ovale, foramen spinosum, emissary sphenoidal foramen (of Vesalius), and the foramen lacerum.

The optic canal links the central area of the middle cranial fossa with the apex of the orbit. It transmits the optic nerve and the ophthalmic artery.

The superior orbital fissure lies between the greater and lesser wings of the sphenoid bone. It is located on the anterior wall of the middle cranial fossa and links the fossa with the apex of the orbit. The fissure transmits many structures. The nerves passing through it are the oculomotor, trochlear and abducent nerves, the lacrimal, frontal and nasociliary branches of the ophthalmic nerve, and filaments from the internal carotid plexus (sympathetic). It also transmits the ophthalmic veins, and the orbital branch of the middle meningeal artery and the recurrent branch of the lacrimal artery.

The foramen rotundum lies within the greater wing of the sphenoid. It allows communication between the lateral part of the middle cranial fossa and the pterygopalatine fossa. Passing through it is the maxillary nerve. The foramen ovale is also present in the greater wing of the sphenoid, but it links the middle cranial fossa to the infratemporal fossa. The major structure passing through it is the mandibular nerve. In addition, there is the lesser petrosal branch of the glossopharyngeal nerve, the accessory meningeal branch of the maxillary artery, and an emissary vein from the cavernous venous sinus to the pterygoid venous plexus in the infratemporal fossa.

The foramen spinosum lies just behind the foramen ovale. It transmits the meningeal branch of the mandibular nerve and the middle meningeal vessels. In front of, and medial to, the foramen ovale is the sphenoidal emissary foramen (of Vesalius). Both the sphenoidal emissary foramen and foramen spinosum link the middle cranial fossa and infratemporal fossa. The sphenoidal emissary foramen is often absent but, when present, it transmits an emissary vein from the cavernous sinus to the pterygoid plexus.

The foramen lacerum lies at the junction between the apex of the petrous process, the sphenoid bone and the basilar part of the occipital bone. Structures associated with the foramen are the internal carotid artery (entering from behind and emerging above), the greater petrosal nerve and the deep petrosal nerve (which join to form the nerve of the pterygoid canal), a meningeal branch of the ascending pharyngeal artery, and emissary veins linking the cavernous sinus and pterygoid venous plexus.

Other features seen on the floor of the middle cranial fossa are the trigeminal impression, hiatuses and grooves for the greater and lesser petrosal nerves, the petrous ridge and arcuate eminence, and grooves for the middle meningeal vessels and the superior petrosal venous sinuses. With the exception of the grooves for the middle meningeal vessels, these features are associated with the petrous part of the temporal bone.

The trigeminal impression is a shallow fossa situated behind the foramen lacerum. It indicates the site of the ganglion of the trigeminal nerve.

The greater and lesser petrosal nerves arise within the temporal bone in the region of the middle ear. They emerge onto the floor of the middle cranial fossa through hiatuses, the hiatus for the lesser petrosal nerve lying lateral to that of the greater petrosal nerve. The groove for the greater petrosal nerve runs forwards from the hiatus to the foramen lacerum. The groove for the lesser petrosal nerve runs forwards from the hiatus towards the foramen ovale.

The petrous ridge marks the boundary between the middle and posterior cranial fossae. A distinct bulge called the arcuate eminence lies on the petrous ridge. This indicates the position of the anterior (superior) semicircular canal of the internal ear. Running along the ridge is the groove for the

superior petrosal venous sinus. This sinus links the cavernous and the sigmoid sinuses.

There is a conspicuous groove for the middle meningeal vessels. This groove runs across the floor of the middle cranial fossa, from the foramen spinosum, and up onto the lateral wall of the fossa, where it may divide into a groove for the frontal branches of the vessels and a groove for the parietal branches.

The Posterior Cranial Fossa

The posterior cranial fossa is the largest of the cranial fossae. It contains the hindbrain. The floor and posterior wall of the posterior cranial fossa are formed mainly by the occipital bone (lateral and lower squamous parts). The anterior wall of the fossa leading up to the middle cranial fossa is formed by the basilar part of the occipital bone, the temporal bones (petrous and mastoid parts) and the sphenoid bone (dorsum sellae and posterior part of the body). The region corresponds extracranially with the posterior zone of the cranial base.

The foramen magnum is the most prominent structure in the floor of the posterior cranial fossa. Passing through the foramen are the medulla oblongata, the vertebral and spinal arteries, the spinal parts of the accessory nerves, and the meningeal branches of the cervical spinal nerves. The hypoglossal canals (anterior condylar canals) and condylar canals (posterior condylar canals) lie close to the foramen magnum. The hypoglossal canal transmits the hypoglossal nerve, the meningeal branch of the ascending pharyngeal artery and an emissary vein linking the basilar plexus intracranially with the internal jugular vein extracranially.

The condylar canal carries an emissary vein between the sigmoid sinus and the occipital veins, and a meningeal branch of the occipital artery.

Other features found in the floor of the fossa are the internal occipital protuberance and crest, and grooves for some of the dural venous sinuses. The internal occipital protuberance lies at the confluence of some venous sinuses. Extending down from the protuberance to the foramen magnum is the internal occipital crest. This crest gives attachment to the falx cerebelli. Grooves are found for the transverse, sigmoid, and superior sagittal sinuses. The occipital sinus may groove the internal occipital crest. The margins of the grooves for the transverse and superior petrosal sinuses provide attachments for the tentorium cerebelli.

That part of the fossa in front of the foramen magnum formed by the basilar part of the occipital bone and by the sphenoid bone is called the clivus. Between the clivus and each petrous process of a temporal bone is the petro-occipital fissure. This fissure is occupied in life by a sliver of cartilage. The posterior end of the fissure is widened to form the jugular foramen. Passing through the jugular foramen is the internal jugular vein as it continues from the sigmoid sinus. In addition, it transmits the glossopharyngeal, vagus and accessory nerves, the inferior petrosal sinus and a meningeal branch of the occipital artery. The inferior petrosal sinus runs from the cavernous sinus to the jugular foramen in a groove closely related to the petro-occipital fissure. The posterior surface of the petrous part of the temporal bone shows an internal acoustic meatus for the passage of the facial and vestibulocochlear nerves into the ear. Behind the opening of the internal acoustic meatus is the opening for the aqueduct of the vestibule of the ear.

FLOOR OF CRANIAL CAVITY

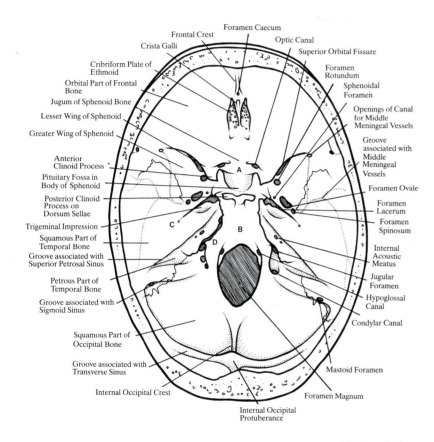

Frontal Crest

Crista Galli

Foramen Caecum

Optic Canal

Superior Orbital Fissure

Cribriform Plate of Ethmoid

Orbital Part of Frontal Bone

Jugum of Sphenoid Bone

Lesser Wing of Sphenoid

Greater Wing of Sphenoid

Foramen Rotundum

Sphenoidal Foramen

Openings of Canal for Middle Meningeal Vessels

Anterior Clinoid Process

Pituitary Fossa in Body of Sphenoid

Posterior Clinoid Process on Dorsum Sellae

Trigeminal Impression

Squamous Part of Temporal Bone

Groove associated with Superior Petrosal Sinus

Petrous Part of Temporal Bone

Groove associated with Sigmoid Sinus

Squamous Part of Occipital Bone

Groove associated with Transverse Sinus

Internal Occipital Crest

Groove associated with Middle Meningeal Vessels

Foramen Ovale

Foramen Lacerum

Foramen Spinosum

Internal Acoustic Meatus

Jugular Foramen

Hypoglossal Canal

Condylar Canal

Mastoid Foramen

Foramen Magnum

Internal Occipital Protuberance

A. Prechiasmatic Groove
B. Basilar Part of Occipital Bone
C. Hiatus and Groove for Greater Petrosal Nerve
D. Petro-occipital Fissure

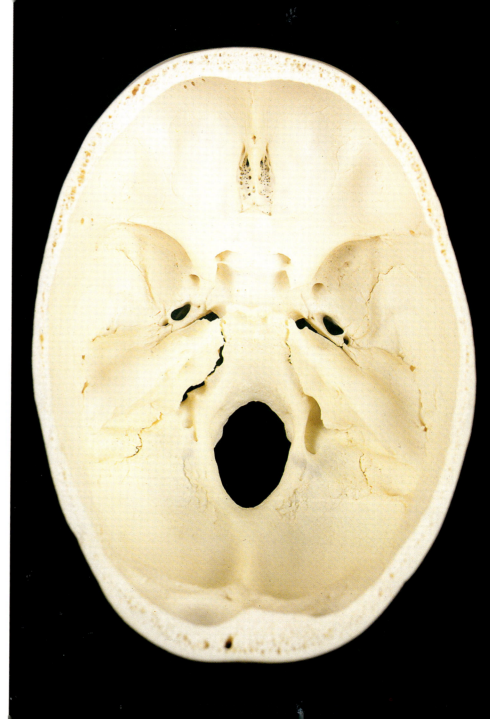

THE NORMA VERTICALIS
(The Calvaria)

The view of the skull from above is so named because the most superior point of the skull is called the vertex. The region observed is the skullcap or calvaria.

The calvaria is approximately oval in shape, the anteroposterior dimension being the greater. It is usually wider posteriorly than anteriorly. It is comprised of four bones separated by three prominent sutures. Anteriorly is found the squamous part of the frontal bone. Posteriorly is the squamous part of the occipital bone. Between the frontal and occipital bones lie the two parietal bones. The suture between the frontal bone and the parietal bones is called the coronal suture. The midline suture between the parietal bones is the sagittal suture. The junction of the coronal and sagittal sutures is termed the bregma. The bregma corresponds to the anterior fontanelle on the fetal skull. The suture dividing the occipital bone from the parietal bones is the lambdoid suture.

The point of meeting of the lambdoid suture and the sagittal suture of the calvaria is termed the lambda. This site marks the position of the posterior fontanelle on the fetal skull.

The calvaria is otherwise rather featureless. The region of maximum convexity of the parietal bone is called the parietal tuberosity. Close to the tuberosity run the superior and inferior temporal lines, though these lines are best seen in the norma lateralis. Parietal foramina may be found on either side of the sagittal suture. They transmit emissary veins from the superior sagittal sinus within the cranium. Sometimes terminal branches of the occipital arteries also pass through the parietal foramina.

The internal surface of the calvaria shows many of the features already described. However, the sutures tend to be less distinct because their gradual obliteration with age begins on the intracranial surface. Additional features seen intracranially include the frontal crest, some grooves for vascular structures and some depressions associated with arachnoid granulations.

The frontal crest is a prominent projection into the cranial cavity anteriorly. It provides attachment for a sheet of meninges, the falx cerebri, which passes between the two cerebral hemispheres of the brain. Running from the frontal crest and across the calvaria in the midline is a groove for the superior sagittal venous sinus. On each side of this groove may be found the depressions for arachnoid granulations. Deep grooves for middle meningeal vessels are often found on the parietal bones.

EXTERNAL VIEW OF CALVARIA

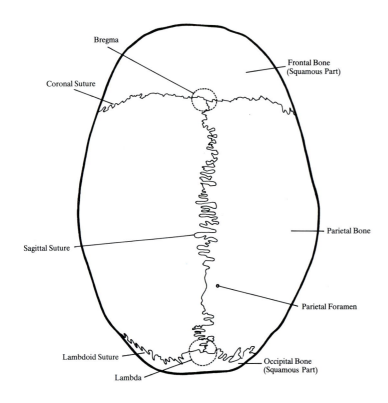

Bregma

Frontal Bone
(Squamous Part)

Coronal Suture

Sagittal Suture

Parietal Bone

Parietal Foramen

Lambdoid Suture

Lambda

Occipital Bone
(Squamous Part)

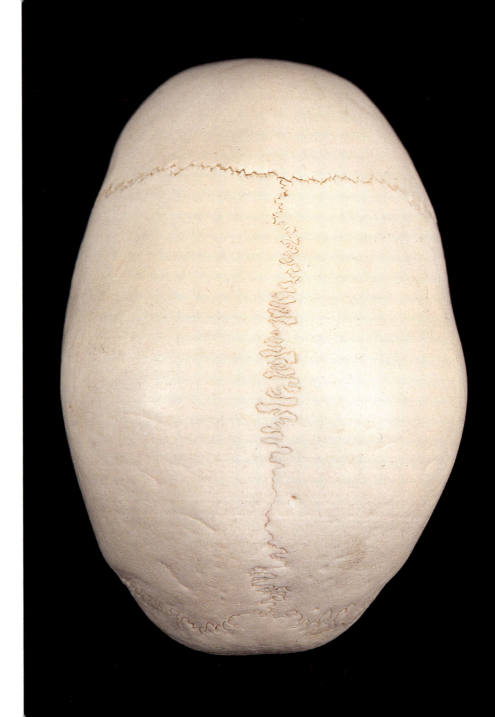

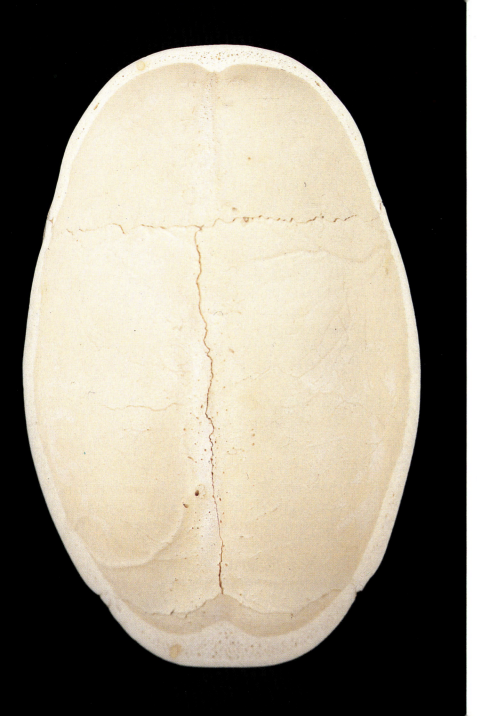

INTERNAL VIEW OF CALVARIA

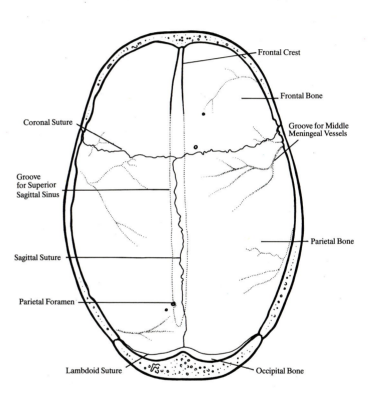

Frontal Crest

Frontal Bone

Groove for Middle Meningeal Vessels

Coronal Suture

Groove for Superior Sagittal Sinus

Parietal Bone

Sagittal Suture

Parietal Foramen

Lambdoid Suture

Occipital Bone

THE ORBIT AND NASAL CAVITY

The Orbit

The upper part of the facial skeleton shows two pyramid-shaped cavities called the orbital cavities (or orbits). They house and protect the eyes and thus should be regarded as part of the neurocranium.

The orbital aperture (aditus of the orbit) is bounded above by the supra-orbital margin of the frontal bone, laterally by the zygomatic bone and the zygomatic process of the frontal bone, below by the zygomatic bone and the maxilla, and medially by the frontal bone and the anterior lacrimal crest of the frontal process of the maxilla.

The orbital cavity is pyramidal in shape, with the apex pointing posteriorly. It has a roof, a floor, and medial and lateral walls. The bones that comprise the orbital cavity are the ethmoid, frontal, lacrimal, maxillary, palatine, sphenoid, and zygomatic bones.

The roof of the orbit is formed mainly by the orbital part of the frontal bone. The lesser wing of the sphenoid bone is situated posteriorly at the apex.

The floor of the orbit is made up of the orbital surfaces of the maxillary and the zygomatic bones, with a small contribution from the palatine bone near the apex (the orbital process of the palatine bone).

The medial wall of the orbit begins at the anterior lacrimal crest of the maxilla. Behind this lies the lacrimal bone. Most of the medial wall behind the lacrimal bone is formed by the orbital plate of the ethmoid bone. The body of the sphenoid bone contributes to the medial wall posteriorly. Between the anterior lacrimal crest of the maxilla and the posterior lacrimal crest of the lacrimal bone is the fossa for the lacrimal sac.

The lateral wall of the orbit is formed anteriorly by the orbital surface of the zygomatic bone, and posteriorly by the orbital surface of the greater wing of the sphenoid bone.

There are several foramina and fissures within the orbit:

At the superior orbital margin are the supra-orbital notch (or foramen) and the frontal notch (or foramen). These transmit respectively the supra-orbital and the supratrochlear nerves and vessels.

In the floor of the orbit is found the infra-orbital groove and the infra-orbital canal for the infra-orbital nerve and vessels.

At the medial wall is situated the opening of the nasolacrimal canal, and the anterior and posterior ethmoidal foramina for the anterior and posterior ethmoidal nerves and vessels. The nasolacrimal canal is located antero-inferiorly, close to the orbital margin. The ethmoidal foramina lie at the junction with the roof of the orbital cavity.

At the lateral wall is the zygomatico-orbital foramen (occasionally foramina). Through this foramen pass the zygomatic branches of the maxillary division of the trigeminal nerve (with accompanying vessels).

Near the apex of the orbital cavity are the optic canal, the superior orbital fissure and the inferior orbital fissure. The optic canal lies within the lesser wing of the sphenoid bone. It transmits the optic nerve and the ophthalmic artery. The superior orbital fissure lies between the greater and lesser wings of the sphenoid, at the junction of the roof and lateral wall of the orbit. It transmits the oculomotor, trochlear, ophthalmic and abducent nerves, together with the ophthalmic veins. The inferior orbital fissure lies at the junction of the lateral wall and floor of the orbit, between the greater wing of the sphenoid and the maxilla. Through this fissure pass the infra-orbital and zygomatic branches of the maxillary division of the trigeminal nerve (with accompanying vessels).

The Nasal Cavity

The part of the nose that projects from the face is called the external nose. The nasal cavity internally is divided into two nasal fossae by the nasal septum. Prominent processes project from the lateral walls of the nasal cavity (the superior, middle and inferior nasal conchae). The lateral walls are also significant for being the sites of drainage of the ethmoidal, frontal, maxillary and sphenoidal air sinuses and of the nasolacrimal ducts.

The anterior nasal aperture (piriform aperture) is bounded mainly by the maxillary bones. The nasal bones form the superior margin of the aperture.

The nasal fossa must remain patent for ventilation. The patency is maintained by the rigidity of the bony walls. Each nasal fossa has a roof, a floor, a lateral wall and a medial wall.

The medial wall is formed by the nasal septum. It comprises the septal cartilage anteriorly, the perpendicular plate of the ethmoid bone posterosuperiorly, and the vomer postero-inferiorly. At the base of the nasal septum is the nasal crest formed by the maxillary and palatine bones.

The bones that comprise the remaining walls of the nasal fossa are the ethmoid, frontal, lacrimal, maxillary, nasal, palatine, sphenoid and vomer, and the bone of the inferior concha.

The roof of the nasal fossa is formed centrally by the cribriform plate of the ethmoid bone. Anteriorly lies the nasal bone and the nasal spine of the frontal bone. Posteriorly is located the body of the sphenoid, overlapped by the ala of the vomer and the sphenoidal process of the palatine bone. The cribriform plate transmits olfactory nerves into the roof of the nasal cavity and also the anterior ethmoidal nerves and vessels.

The floor of the nasal fossa is formed by the palatine process of the maxilla anteriorly and the horizontal plate of the palatine bone posteriorly.

The lateral wall of the nasal fossa consists mainly of the medial surface of the maxilla, with the large maxillary hiatus being reduced in size by the overlapping of the lacrimal and ethmoid bones above, the palatine bone behind and the inferior concha below. From the lateral wall project the three nasal conchae. The superior and middle conchae are part of the labyrinth of the ethmoid bone. The inferior concha is a separate bone. The region above and behind the superior nasal concha is called the spheno-ethmoidal recess. The region between the superior and middle nasal conchae is the superior meatus. Between the middle and inferior conchae is located the middle meatus. Below the inferior nasal concha is the inferior meatus.

The nasolacrimal canal on the lateral wall of the nasal fossa is formed by the lacrimal groove of the maxilla articulating with the descending process of the lacrimal bone and the lacrimal process of the inferior concha.

The sphenopalatine foramen, which links the nasal cavity with the pterygopalatine fossa, lies high up in the posterior part of the lateral wall. It is formed by the notch between the orbital and sphenoidal processes of the perpendicular plate of the palatine bone articulating with the body of the sphenoid bone. This foramen transmits the nasopalatine and posterior superior nasal nerves and the sphenopalatine vessels.

The lateral wall of the nose is noted for being the site of drainage of the paranasal air sinuses. The sphenoidal sinus drains into the spheno-ethmoidal recess. The posterior ethmoidal air cells drain into the superior meatus. The frontal and maxillary air sinuses and the anterior and middle ethmoidal air cells drain into the middle meatus. The opening of the nasolacrimal canal lies in the inferior meatus.

The posterior nasal apertures (choanae) link the nasal fossae with the nasopharynx. The bones that contribute to this region are the palatine, sphenoid and vomer bones. The posterior border of the vomer separates the two posterior nasal apertures. Each aperture is bounded below by the posterior border of the horizontal plate of the palatine bone, laterally by the medial pterygoid plate, and above by the body and vaginal process of the sphenoid bone and the ala of the vomer.

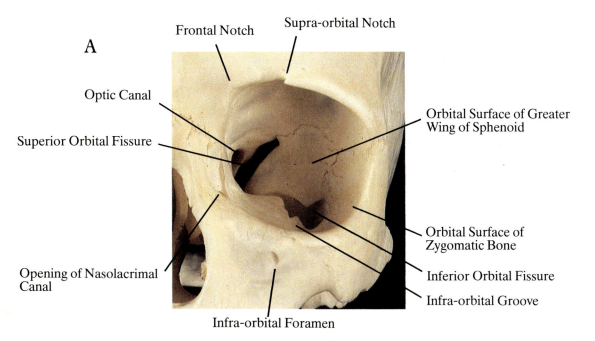

A

Frontal Notch

Supra-orbital Notch

Optic Canal

Superior Orbital Fissure

Orbital Surface of Greater Wing of Sphenoid

Orbital Surface of Zygomatic Bone

Inferior Orbital Fissure

Infra-orbital Groove

Opening of Nasolacrimal Canal

Infra-orbital Foramen

A LATERAL WALL OF ORBIT

B MEDIAL WALL OF ORBIT

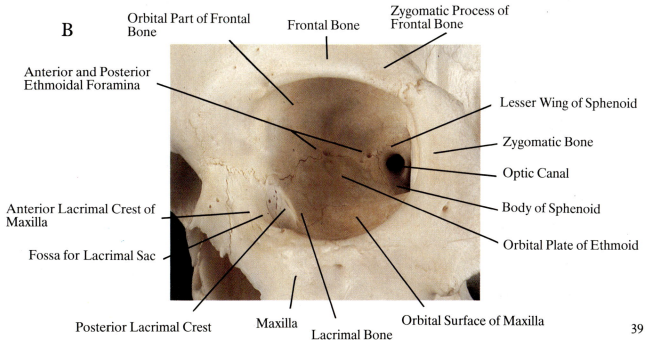

B

Orbital Part of Frontal Bone

Frontal Bone

Zygomatic Process of Frontal Bone

Anterior and Posterior Ethmoidal Foramina

Lesser Wing of Sphenoid

Zygomatic Bone

Optic Canal

Body of Sphenoid

Anterior Lacrimal Crest of Maxilla

Orbital Plate of Ethmoid

Fossa for Lacrimal Sac

Posterior Lacrimal Crest

Maxilla

Lacrimal Bone

Orbital Surface of Maxilla

39

NASAL SEPTUM

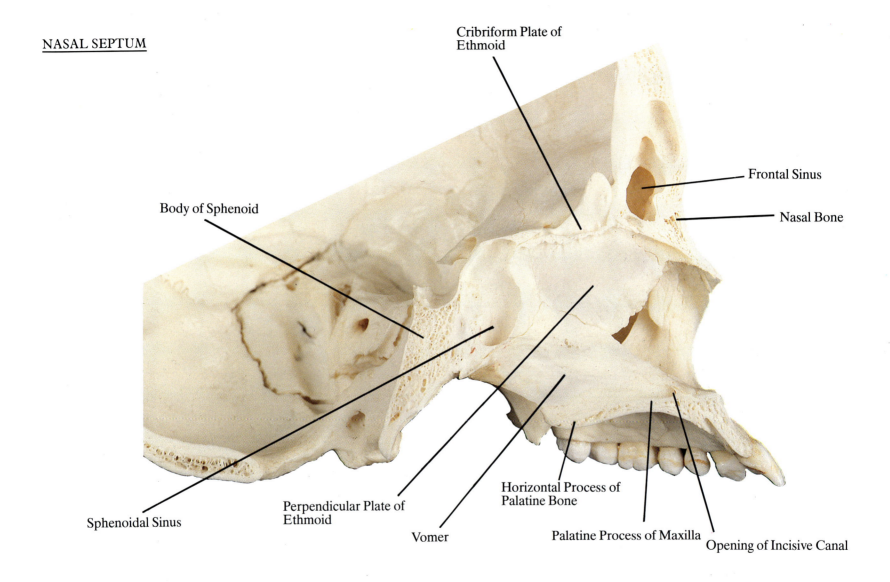

Cribriform Plate of Ethmoid

Frontal Sinus

Nasal Bone

Body of Sphenoid

Sphenoidal Sinus

Perpendicular Plate of Ethmoid

Vomer

Horizontal Process of Palatine Bone

Palatine Process of Maxilla

Opening of Incisive Canal

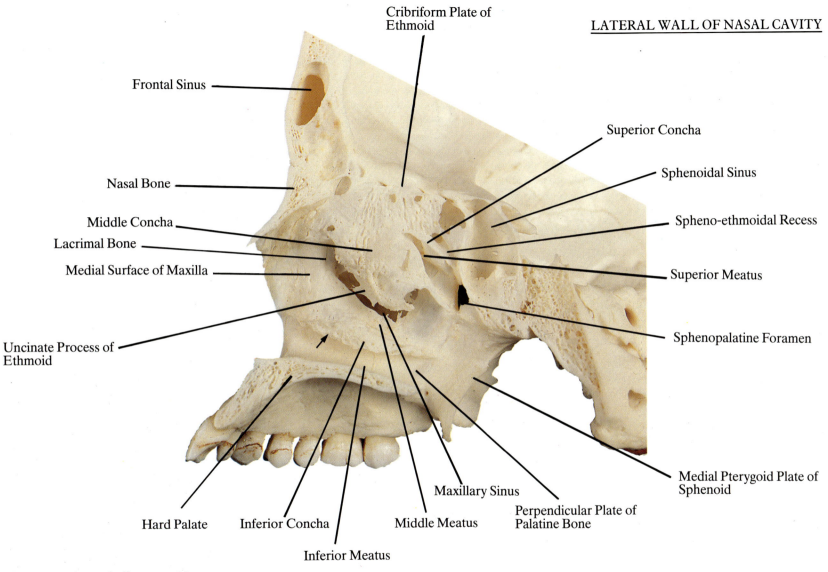

Cribriform Plate of
Ethmoid

Frontal Sinus

Superior Concha

Sphenoidal Sinus

Nasal Bone

Spheno-ethmoidal Recess

Middle Concha

Lacrimal Bone

Superior Meatus

Medial Surface of Maxilla

Sphenopalatine Foramen

Uncinate Process of
Ethmoid

Medial Pterygoid Plate of
Sphenoid

Hard Palate   Inferior Concha   Middle Meatus   Maxillary Sinus

Perpendicular Plate of
Palatine Bone

Inferior Meatus

Arrow indicates position
of opening of
Nasolacrimal canal

THE PARANASAL AIR SINUSES

The paranasal air sinuses are invaginations from the lateral wall of the nose extending into the surrounding bones. There are four sets of paired sinuses: frontal, ethmoidal, sphenoidal and maxillary. There is considerable variation in the morphology of the sinuses from individual to individual, and between the sinuses of each side. The precise function of the paranasal sinuses is unknown, although some believe that the sinuses lighten the skull and add resonance to the voice. It is conceivable, however, that they simply reflect the considerable growth of the bones in which they are situated.

The Frontal Air Sinuses

The frontal sinuses lie in the frontal bone above and behind the superciliary arches. The frontal sinuses are frequently of unequal size, the larger sinus sometimes extending across the midline. The bony septum separating the frontal sinuses is also often asymmetrically positioned. Each sinus may be partially subdivided by additional septa. The anterior ethmoidal air cells may encroach into the frontal sinuses.

The frontal sinus drains into the middle meatus of the lateral wall of the nasal fossa, either through a simple opening or as a channel called the frontonasal duct.

The Ethmoidal Air Sinuses

The ethmoidal air sinuses occupy the two lateral masses (labyrinths) of the ethmoid bone between the lateral wall of the nose and the medial wall of the orbit. The orbital wall is particularly thin.

The walls of the ethmoidal air sinuses are incomplete and are covered by adjacent bones (i.e. frontal, lacrimal, maxillary, sphenoidal and palatine bones). Furthermore, the sinuses may not be restricted to the ethmoid bone, but may encroach into the frontal, maxillary and sphenoidal air sinuses and into the middle nasal concha, uncinate process and agger nasi of the nose.

Each sinus is subdivided into a number of air cells. The air cells are separated from each other by thin, incomplete, bony septa. Three groups of air cells are usually found: anterior, middle and posterior air cells.

The anterior ethmoidal cells occupy the anterior portion of the lateral mass of the ethmoid bone. There are approximately 11 air cells in this group. They drain into the middle meatus of the lateral wall of the nose via the frontonasal duct or the ethmoidal infundibulum.

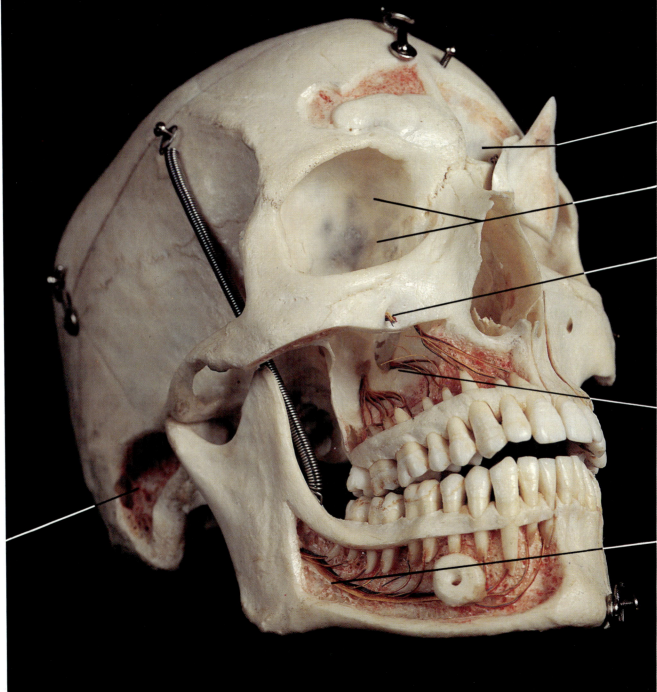

Frontal Sinus

Position of Ethmoidal Air
Cells beneath Orbital Plate
of Ethmoid Bone

Infra-orbital Nerve
emerging after passing
across Roof of Maxillary
Sinus

Maxillary Sinus showing
course of Superior Alveolar
Nerves

Mastoid Antrum

Inferior Alveolar Nerve
within Mandibular Canal

The middle ethmoidal cells produce the ethmoidal bulla in the middle meatus of the lateral wall of the nose. There are usually three middle ethmoidal air cells. They drain on or above the bulla.

There are about six posterior ethmoidal cells. They lie in the posterior portion of the lateral mass of the ethmoid bone. They drain into the superior meatus of the lateral wall of the nose.

The Sphenoidal Air Sinuses

These two sinuses lie within the body of the sphenoid bone at the back of the nasal cavity. They are separated by a bony septum, which is usually positioned asymmetrically. The size of the sinuses varies considerably. Although usually limited to the body of the sphenoid, the sinuses can be found within the greater wings and pterygoid processes of the sphenoid, and even within the basilar part of the occipital bone. Occasionally, a posterior ethmoidal air cell may be found extending into the body of the sphenoid bone.

The sphenoidal sinus drains into the posterior wall of the spheno-ethmoidal recess.

The Maxillary Air Sinuses

These are the largest of the paranasal sinuses. They are situated in the bodies of the maxillary bones.

The maxillary sinus is pyramidal in shape. The base (medial wall) forms part of the lateral wall of the nose. The apex extends into the zygomatic process of the maxilla. The roof of the sinus is part of the floor of the orbit. The floor of the sinus is formed by the alveolar process and part of the palatine process of the maxilla. The anterior wall of the maxillary sinus is the facial surface of the maxilla and the posterior wall is the infratemporal surface of the maxilla. The sinus may be partially divided by incomplete bony septa.

The medial wall of the maxillary sinus has the opening (ostium) of the sinus. The roof has the infra-orbital nerve and vessels within the infra-orbital canal. The floor of the sinus is related to the roots of the cheek teeth. The anterior superior alveolar nerve and vessels (which arise from the infra-orbital nerve and vessels near the midpoint of the infra-orbital canal) pass downwards in a fine canal (canalis sinuosus) in the anterior wall of the maxillary sinus to be distributed to the anterior teeth. The posterior superior alveolar nerve and vessels pass through canals in the posterior surface of the sinus. The middle superior alveolar nerve is found in about 70 per cent of subjects. It may run in the posterior, lateral or anterior walls of the maxillary sinus to terminate at the premolar teeth.

In an isolated maxillary bone, the ostium of the maxillary sinus is large. However, the ostium in an intact specimen is considerably reduced by portions of the adjacent bones (namely the perpendicular plate of the palatine bone, the uncinate process of the ethmoid bone, the inferior nasal concha and the lacrimal bone) and by the overlying nasal mucosa. The ostium lies high up at the back of the medial wall of the maxillary sinus, being unfavourably situated for drainage. It usually opens into the posterior part of the ethmoidal infundibulum, and hence into the hiatus semilunaris of the lateral wall of the nose. An accessory ostium is sometimes present behind the major ostium.

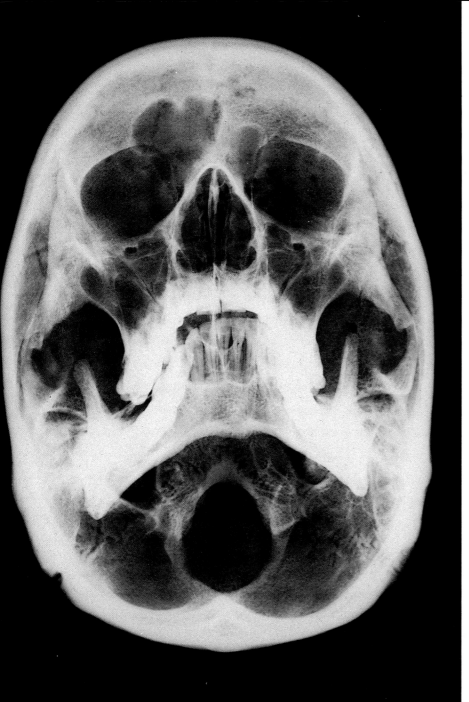

OCCIPITOMENTAL RADIOGRAPH OF SKULL

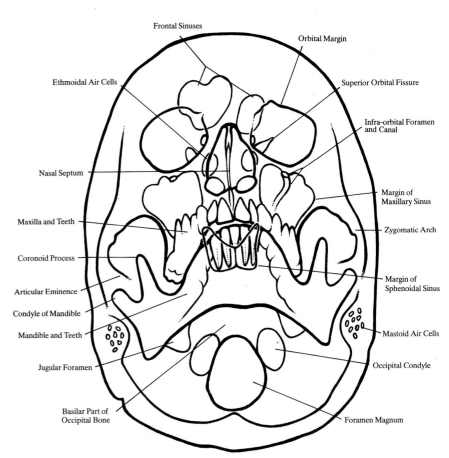

Frontal Sinuses

Orbital Margin

Ethmoidal Air Cells

Superior Orbital Fissure

Infra-orbital Foramen and Canal

Nasal Septum

Margin of Maxillary Sinus

Maxilla and Teeth

Zygomatic Arch

Coronoid Process

Margin of Sphenoidal Sinus

Articular Eminence

Condyle of Mandible

Mandible and Teeth

Mastoid Air Cells

Jugular Foramen

Occipital Condyle

Basilar Part of Occipital Bone

Foramen Magnum

45

THE FETAL SKULL

The skull of a full-term fetus contains the same individual bones as the adult skull. There are, however, significant differences with respect to the proportions of the skull, the size and shape of the bones, and the way the bones articulate.

Considering the proportions of the fetal skull, the neurocranium is much larger than the viscerocranium. Indeed, the ratio of the neurocranium to the viscerocranium is 8:1 for the fetal skull and only 3:1 for the adult skull. Thus, whereas the neurocranium expands much faster during the fetal period, the face grows predominantly in the years after birth. This relates to the fact that early in development the brain causes the neurocranium to expand, but later, structures such as the teeth and the jaw musculature are responsible for significant growth of the face. There is thus differential growth in the transformation of the fetal to the adult skull.

The individual bones of the fetal skull are obviously smaller than their adult counterparts, the exceptions being the ear ossicles (malleus, incus and stapes), which have almost reached adult size by birth. In addition, many of the bones have slightly different shapes, mainly because of the different proportions of their constituent parts. The bones comprising the cranial vault are more curved and the frontal and parietal tuberosities are especially prominent. The superciliary arches and the glabella on the frontal bone have not developed. The temporal bone has only a rudimentary mastoid process and the stylomastoid foramen is therefore superficial. The mandibular fossa is flat and there is no articular tubercle. The external acoustic meatus is short and the future bony part is unossified. Consequently, the tympanic membrane is relatively superficial. For the ethmoid bone, only the labyrinths are ossified at birth. The fetal mandible has no mental protuberance and has a body that is large compared with the ramus. Most of the body is comprised of the alveolar process containing the developing teeth. Each maxillary bone also consists mainly of its alveolar process. The palate is shallow.

Concerning the articulations of the fetal skull, the prominent feature is the presence of six fontanelles. These are fibrous membranes that fill in deficiencies between the bones of the vault of the skull. The fontanelles permit some sliding of the bones of the cranium during passage of the head through the birth canal. At the top of the cranium are the anterior and posterior fontanelles. The anterior fontanelle is the largest of all the fontanelles and is diamond-shaped. It lies between the frontal bone and the parietal bones and corresponds with the bregma of the adult skull. The posterior fontanelle is small and triangular. It corresponds with the lambda, being situated between the occipital bone and the parietal bones. On each side of the skull are found a sphenoidal (anterolateral) fontanelle and a mastoid (posterolateral) fontanelle. Both are small and irregular in shape. The sphenoidal fontanelle corresponds to the pterion of the adult skull. The mastoid fontanelle corresponds to the asterion. The posterior and sphenoidal fontanelles close within three months of birth. The mastoid fontanelle closes at 12 months. The anterior fontanelle is the last to close, at about 18 months.

The sutures on the fetal skull are smooth and wide. There are also sutures and other joints that are usually absent on the adult skull. These exist where parts of a bone have not yet fused to form a single bone.

Dividing the frontal bone down the middle of the forehead is the frontal or metopic suture. Its presence is responsible for the large size and diamond shape of the anterior fontanelle. The frontal suture usually disappears by the age of seven years.

Also in the midline, separating the two halves of the mandible, is the mandibular symphysis (symphysis menti). The mandible becomes a single bone by the age of two years.

The occipital bone at birth is divided into four parts corresponding to the squamous, basilar and lateral parts of the adult bone. Complete fusion takes place by the age of six years. At the junction of the basilar part of the occipital bone and the body of the sphenoid bone is the spheno-occipital synchondrosis. This joint is important for growth of the skull in the anteroposterior plane. It closes at about 20 years of age.

The sphenoid bone at birth has three parts: a central part (the body and lesser wings) and two lateral components (the greater wing and pterygoid process on each side). These unite by the first year.

The temporal bone at birth has three parts. These correspond to the petrous part, the squamous/tympanic part, and the styloid process of the adult bone. Union commences at birth and is complete by the end of the first year. The tip of the styloid process does not, however, fuse with the rest of the bone until at least puberty.

The ethmoid bone is also in three parts: the ethmoid labyrinths laterally and the cribriform and perpendicular plates centrally. Only the labyrinths have begun to ossify by birth. The three parts of the ethmoid fuse to form a single bone at about the age of two years.

The air sinuses within the fetal skull are poorly developed. The maxillary sinus is rudimentary at birth, although it is identifiable radiographically. The sphenoidal sinuses and the ethmoidal air cells may also have reached a sufficient size to be of clinical significance. The frontal sinuses, however, do not invade the frontal bone until the age of two years.

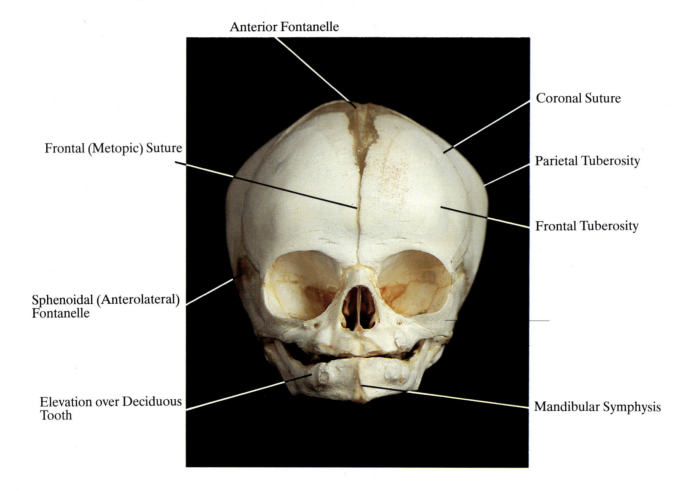

Anterior Fontanelle

Coronal Suture

Parietal Tuberosity

Frontal (Metopic) Suture

Frontal Tuberosity

Sphenoidal (Anterolateral)
Fontanelle

Elevation over Deciduous
Tooth

Mandibular Symphysis

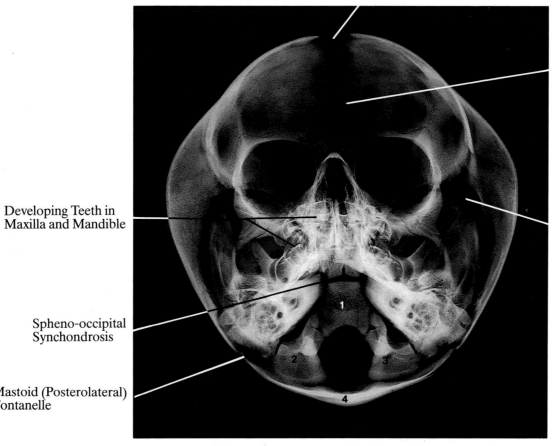

Anterior Fontanelle

Frontal (Metopic) Suture

Developing Teeth in
Maxilla and Mandible

Sphenoidal (Anterolateral)
Fontanelle

Spheno-occipital
Synchondrosis

Mastoid (Posterolateral)
Fontanelle

1 → 4: Four Parts of
Occipital Bone disposed
around Foramen Magnum

NORMA LATERALIS OF NEONATAL SKULL

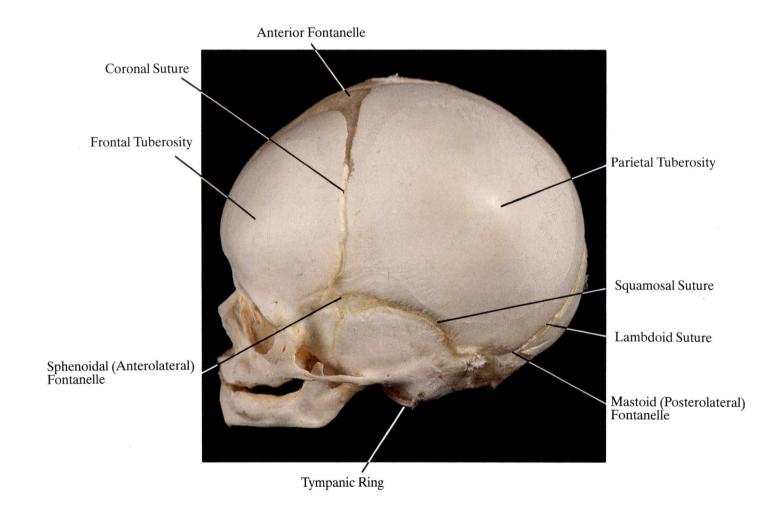

Anterior Fontanelle

Coronal Suture

Frontal Tuberosity

Parietal Tuberosity

Squamosal Suture

Lambdoid Suture

Sphenoidal (Anterolateral)
Fontanelle

Mastoid (Posterolateral)
Fontanelle

Tympanic Ring

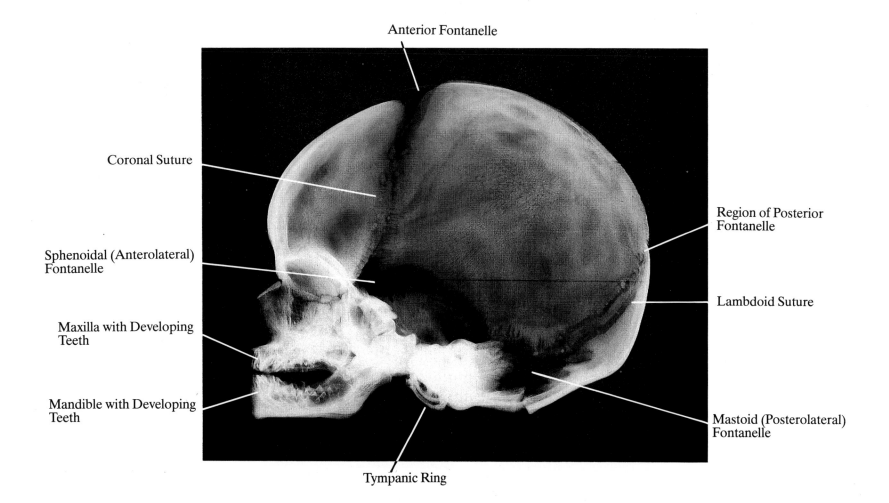

Anterior Fontanelle

Coronal Suture

Region of Posterior
Fontanelle

Sphenoidal (Anterolateral)
Fontanelle

Lambdoid Suture

Maxilla with Developing
Teeth

Mandible with Developing
Teeth

Mastoid (Posterolateral)
Fontanelle

Tympanic Ring

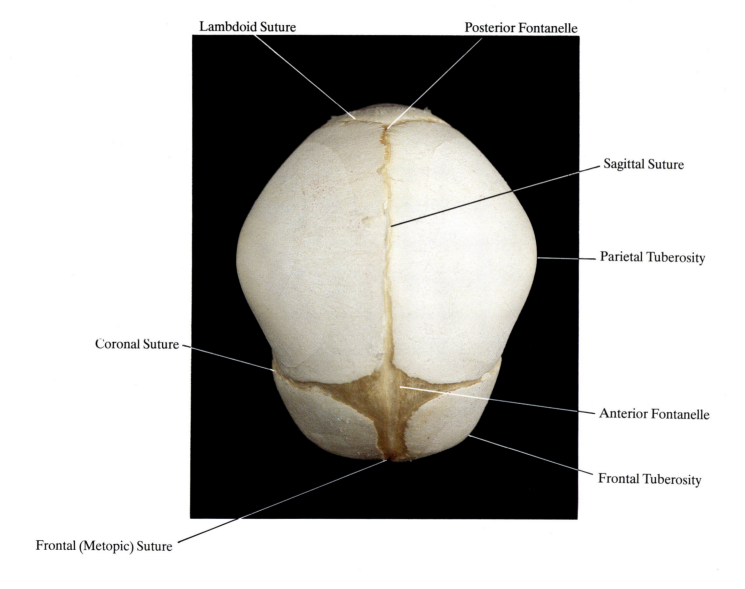

Lambdoid Suture

Posterior Fontanelle

Sagittal Suture

Parietal Tuberosity

Coronal Suture

Anterior Fontanelle

Frontal Tuberosity

Frontal (Metopic) Suture

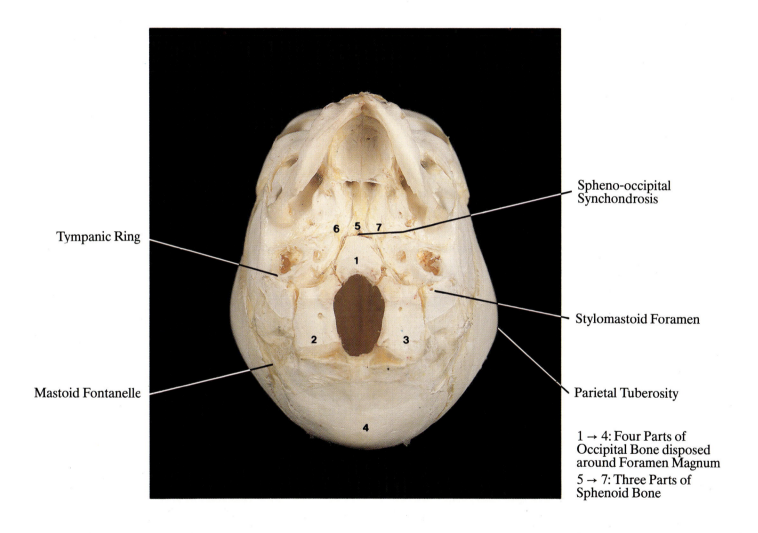

Spheno-occipital
Synchondrosis

Tympanic Ring

Stylomastoid Foramen

Mastoid Fontanelle

Parietal Tuberosity

1 → 4: Four Parts of
Occipital Bone disposed
around Foramen Magnum

5 → 7: Three Parts of
Sphenoid Bone

INDIVIDUAL BONES OF THE SKULL

NAME	NUMBER	PRIMARY LOCATION	SHORT DESCRIPTION	MAIN PARTS	OSSIFICATION
FRONTAL	1	Cranial vault	Forms forehead and roof of orbital cavities	Squamous; nasal; orbital	Intramembranous, two centres
PARIETAL	2	Cranial vault	Forms mid-portion of cranial vault	—	Intramembranous, two centres
OCCIPITAL	1	Cranial vault	Forms back of head. Also contributes to cranial base	Squamous; basilar; lateral	Intramembranous and endochondral, seven centres
ETHMOID	1	Nasal and orbital cavities of face	T-shaped. Processes form superior and middle conchae of lateral wall of nasal cavities	Perpendicular plate; cribriform plate; ethmoidal labyrinths	Endochondrally, three centres
SPHENOID	1	Cranial base	Butterfly-shaped. Also contributes to orbital and nasal cavities and to lateral sides of skull	Body; lesser and greater wings; pterygoid processes	Intramembranous and endochondral, 14 centres
TEMPORAL	2	Cranial base	Also contributes to lateral sides of skull	Squamous; tympanic; petrous (including mastoid); styloid process	Intramembranous and endochondral, eight centres
MALLEUS	2	Acoustic cavity	Shaped like a hammer	Head; neck; handle; anterior and lateral process	Endochondral and intramembranous, two centres

NAME	NUMBER	PRIMARY LOCATION	SHORT DESCRIPTION	MAIN PARTS	OSSIFICATION
INCUS	2	Acoustic cavity	Shaped like an anvil	Body; long and short limbs	Endochondral, single centre
STAPES	2	Acoustic cavity	Stirrup-shaped	Head; neck; two limbs; base	Endochondral, single centre
MANDIBLE	1	Jaws	Forms lower jaw	Body; ramus; alveolar, condylar and coronoid processes	Intramembranous, single centre (secondary cartilages)
MAXILLA	2	Jaws	Forms upper jaw. Also contributes to nasal and orbital cavities	Body; frontal, zygomatic, palatine and alveolar processes	Intramembranous, single centre
PALATINE	2	Nasal cavity of face	L-shaped. Contributes to lateral wall of nose and hard palate	Perpendicular plate; horizontal plate; pyramidal process	Intramembranous, single centre
ZYGOMATIC	2	Face	Forms cheek bone	Body; frontal process; temporal process; orbital plate	Intramembranous, single centre
INFERIOR CONCHA	2	Nasal cavity of face	Projects from lateral wall of nasal cavity	Body; lacrimal, ethmoid and maxillary processes	Endochrondral, single centre
NASAL	2	Face	Forms bridge of nose	—	Intramembranous, single centre
VOMER	1	Nasal cavity of face	Contributes to nasal septum. Plough-shaped	Body; alae	Intramembranous, two centres
LACRIMAL	2	Orbital cavity of face	Situated on medial wall of orbital cavity. Related to lacrimal sac	—	Intramembranous, single centre

● *In the illustrations of individual bones which follow, where paired, the left bone is illustrated.*

A

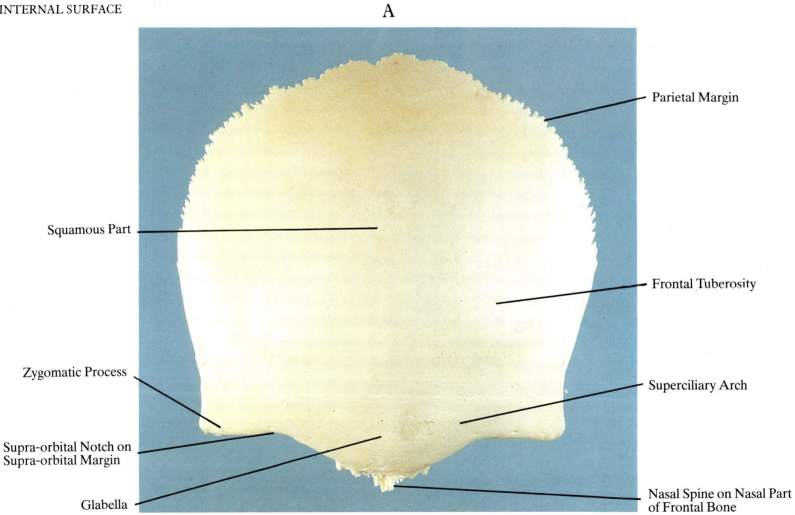

Parietal Margin

Squamous Part

Frontal Tuberosity

Zygomatic Process

Superciliary Arch

Supra-orbital Notch on
Supra-orbital Margin

Glabella

Nasal Spine on Nasal Part
of Frontal Bone

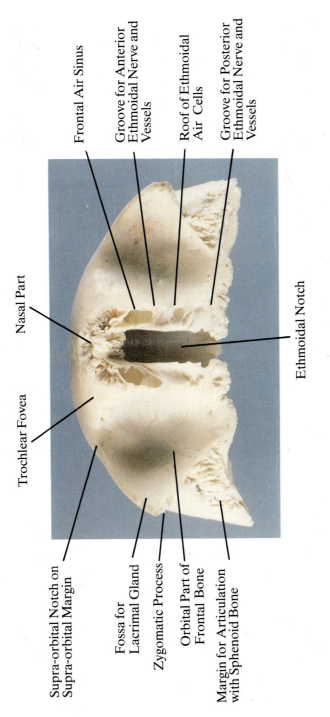

B

Supra-orbital Notch on
Supra-orbital Margin

Fossa for
Lacrimal Gland

Zygomatic Process

Orbital Part of
Frontal Bone

Margin for Articulation
with Sphenoid Bone

Trochlear Fovea

Nasal Part

Frontal Air Sinus

Groove for Anterior
Ethmoidal Nerve and
Vessels

Roof of Ethmoidal
Air Cells

Groove for Posterior
Ethmoidal Nerve and
Vessels

Ethmoidal Notch

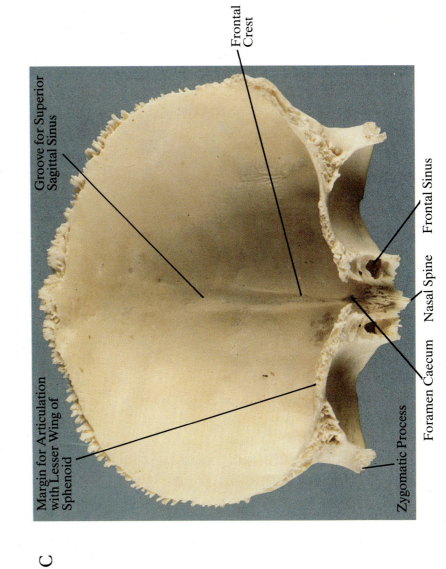

C

Groove for Superior
Sagittal Sinus

Margin for Articulation
with Lesser Wing of
Sphenoid

Frontal
Crest

Frontal Sinus

Nasal Spine

Foramen Caecum

Zygomatic Process

A EXTERNAL SURFACE
B INTERNAL SURFACE

A

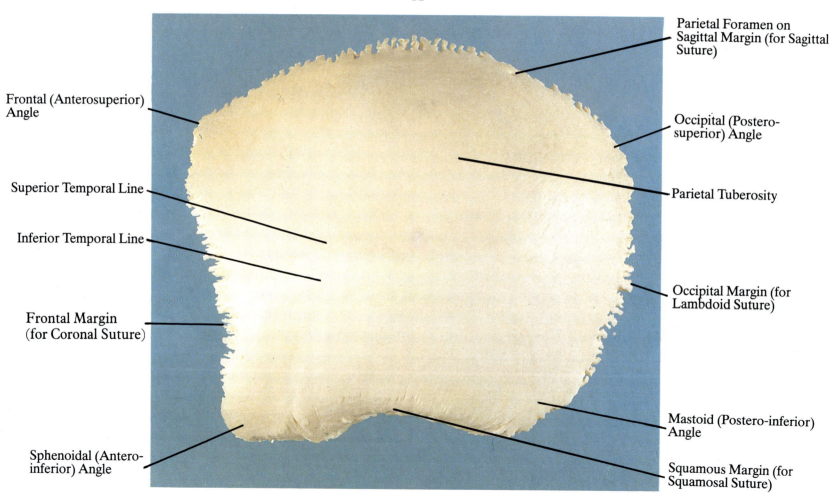

Parietal Foramen on Sagittal Margin (for Sagittal Suture)

Frontal (Anterosuperior) Angle

Occipital (Postero-superior) Angle

Superior Temporal Line

Parietal Tuberosity

Inferior Temporal Line

Frontal Margin (for Coronal Suture)

Occipital Margin (for Lambdoid Suture)

Sphenoidal (Antero-inferior) Angle

Mastoid (Postero-inferior) Angle

Squamous Margin (for Squamosal Suture)

B

Parietal Foramen

Groove for Superior
Sagittal Sinus

Groove for Middle
Meningeal Vessels

Groove for Sigmoid Sinus

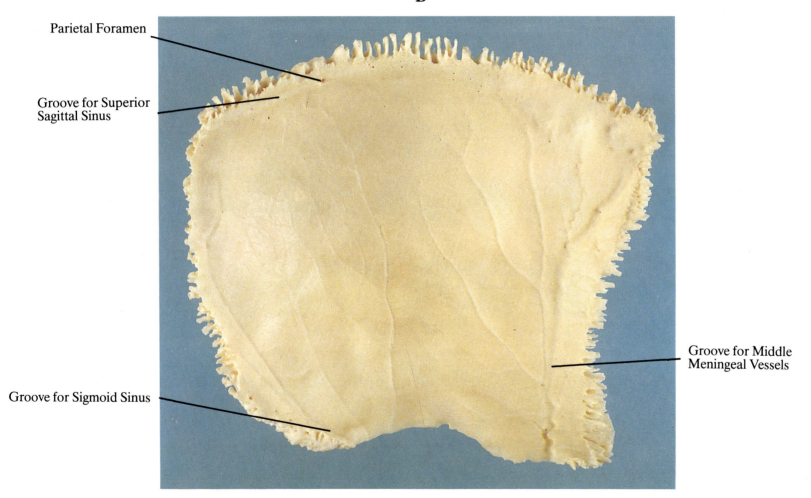

A POSTERIOR VIEW
B INFERIOR VIEW
C and D INTERNAL SURFACE

A

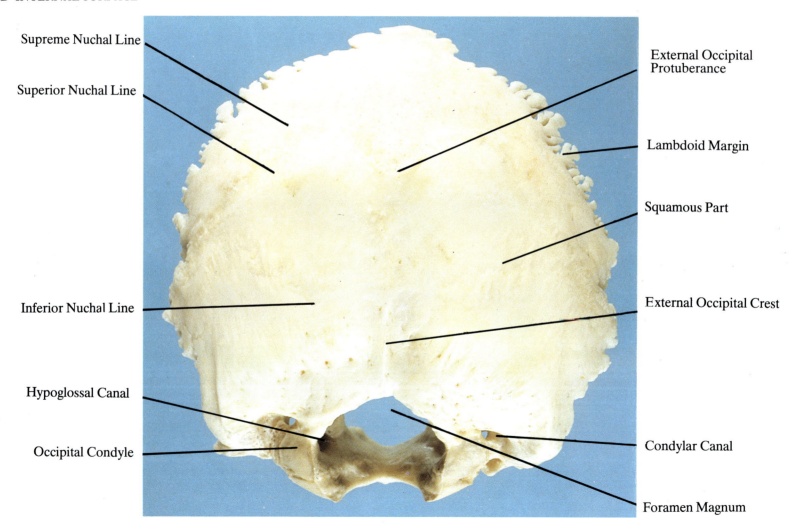

Supreme Nuchal Line

Superior Nuchal Line

Inferior Nuchal Line

Hypoglossal Canal

Occipital Condyle

External Occipital Protuberance

Lambdoid Margin

Squamous Part

External Occipital Crest

Condylar Canal

Foramen Magnum

B

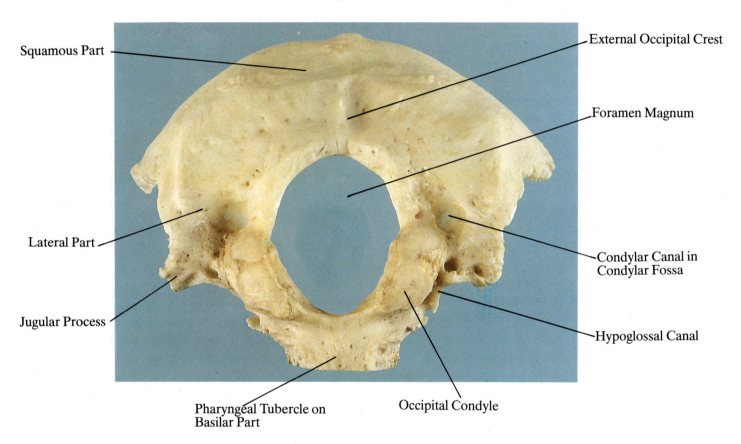

Squamous Part

External Occipital Crest

Foramen Magnum

Lateral Part

Condylar Canal in
Condylar Fossa

Jugular Process

Hypoglossal Canal

Pharyngeal Tubercle on
Basilar Part

Occipital Condyle

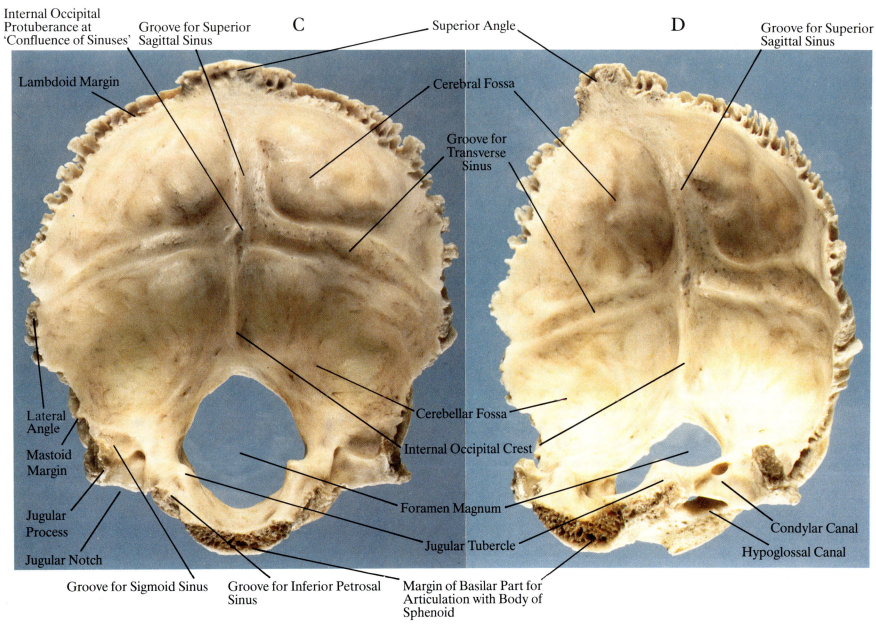

Internal Occipital
Protuberance at
'Confluence of Sinuses'

Groove for Superior
Sagittal Sinus

C

Superior Angle

D

Groove for Superior
Sagittal Sinus

Lambdoid Margin

Cerebral Fossa

Groove for
Transverse
Sinus

Lateral
Angle

Mastoid
Margin

Jugular
Process

Cerebellar Fossa

Internal Occipital Crest

Jugular Notch

Foramen Magnum

Condylar Canal

Hypoglossal Canal

Groove for Sigmoid Sinus

Groove for Inferior Petrosal
Sinus

Jugular Tubercle

Margin of Basilar Part for
Articulation with Body of
Sphenoid

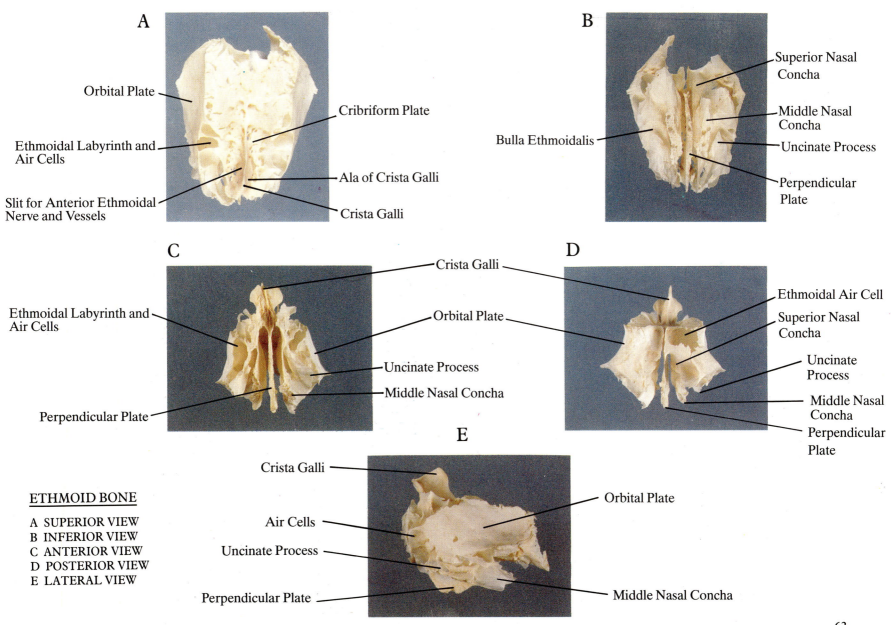

A

Orbital Plate

Ethmoidal Labyrinth and
Air Cells

Slit for Anterior Ethmoidal
Nerve and Vessels

Cribriform Plate

Ala of Crista Galli

Crista Galli

B

Superior Nasal
Concha

Middle Nasal
Concha

Uncinate Process

Bulla Ethmoidalis

Perpendicular
Plate

C

Ethmoidal Labyrinth and
Air Cells

Perpendicular Plate

Crista Galli

Orbital Plate

Uncinate Process

Middle Nasal Concha

D

Crista Galli

Ethmoidal Air Cell

Superior Nasal
Concha

Uncinate
Process

Middle Nasal
Concha

Perpendicular
Plate

E

Crista Galli

Air Cells

Uncinate Process

Perpendicular Plate

Orbital Plate

Middle Nasal Concha

ETHMOID BONE

A SUPERIOR VIEW
B INFERIOR VIEW
C ANTERIOR VIEW
D POSTERIOR VIEW
E LATERAL VIEW

63

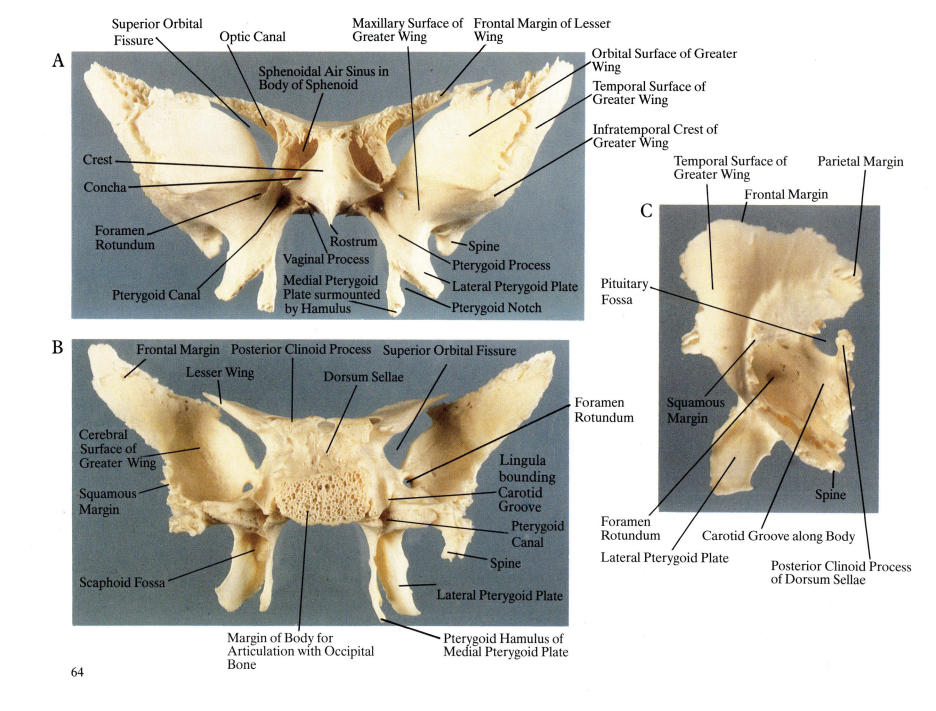

A

Superior Orbital Fissure

Optic Canal

Maxillary Surface of Greater Wing

Frontal Margin of Lesser Wing

Orbital Surface of Greater Wing

Temporal Surface of Greater Wing

Infratemporal Crest of Greater Wing

Sphenoidal Air Sinus in Body of Sphenoid

Crest

Concha

Foramen Rotundum

Rostrum

Vaginal Process

Medial Pterygoid Plate surmounted by Hamulus

Spine

Pterygoid Process

Lateral Pterygoid Plate

Pterygoid Notch

Pterygoid Canal

B

Frontal Margin

Lesser Wing

Posterior Clinoid Process

Dorsum Sellae

Superior Orbital Fissure

Cerebral Surface of Greater Wing

Foramen Rotundum

Lingula bounding Carotid Groove

Squamous Margin

Pterygoid Canal

Spine

Scaphoid Fossa

Lateral Pterygoid Plate

Margin of Body for Articulation with Occipital Bone

Pterygoid Hamulus of Medial Pterygoid Plate

C

Temporal Surface of Greater Wing

Frontal Margin

Parietal Margin

Pituitary Fossa

Squamous Margin

Foramen Rotundum

Lateral Pterygoid Plate

Carotid Groove along Body

Spine

Posterior Clinoid Process of Dorsum Sellae

64

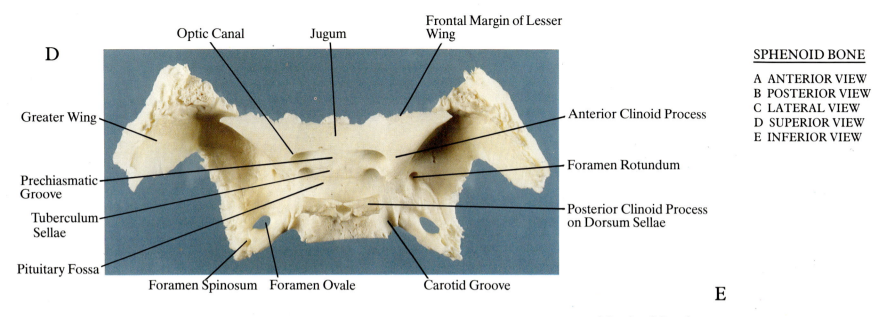

D

Optic Canal

Jugum

Frontal Margin of Lesser Wing

Greater Wing

Anterior Clinoid Process

Prechiasmatic Groove

Foramen Rotundum

Tuberculum Sellae

Posterior Clinoid Process on Dorsum Sellae

Pituitary Fossa

Foramen Spinosum

Foramen Ovale

Carotid Groove

SPHENOID BONE

A ANTERIOR VIEW
B POSTERIOR VIEW
C LATERAL VIEW
D SUPERIOR VIEW
E INFERIOR VIEW

E

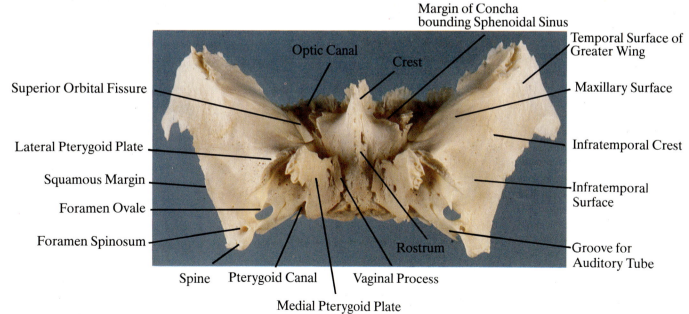

Margin of Concha bounding Sphenoidal Sinus

Optic Canal

Crest

Temporal Surface of Greater Wing

Superior Orbital Fissure

Maxillary Surface

Lateral Pterygoid Plate

Infratemporal Crest

Squamous Margin

Infratemporal Surface

Foramen Ovale

Foramen Spinosum

Rostrum

Groove for Auditory Tube

Spine

Pterygoid Canal

Vaginal Process

Medial Pterygoid Plate

TEMPORAL BONE

A LATERAL VIEW
B POSTERIOR VIEW
C INFERIOR VIEW
D INTERNAL SURFACE

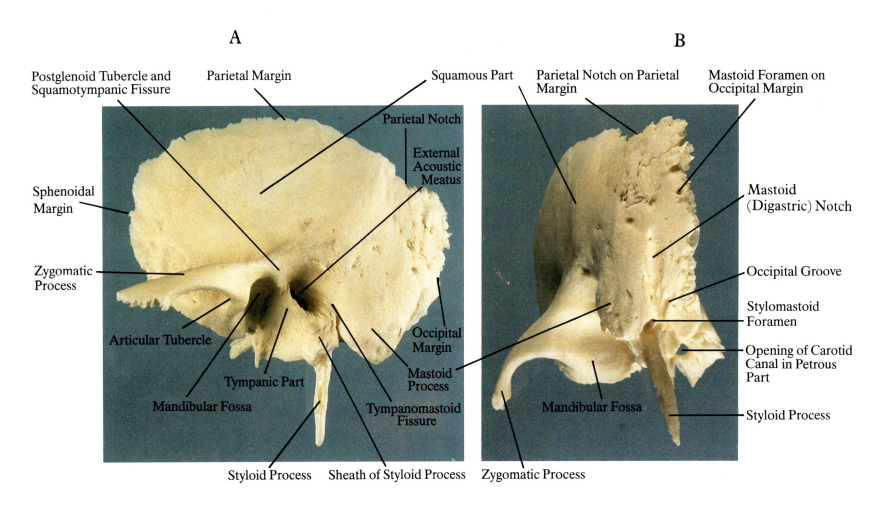

A

Postglenoid Tubercle and Squamotympanic Fissure

Parietal Margin

Squamous Part

Parietal Notch

External Acoustic Meatus

Sphenoidal Margin

Zygomatic Process

Articular Tubercle

Tympanic Part

Occipital Margin

Mandibular Fossa

Mastoid Process

Styloid Process

Tympanomastoid Fissure

Sheath of Styloid Process

B

Parietal Notch on Parietal Margin

Mastoid Foramen on Occipital Margin

Mastoid (Digastric) Notch

Occipital Groove

Stylomastoid Foramen

Opening of Carotid Canal in Petrous Part

Styloid Process

Mandibular Fossa

Zygomatic Process

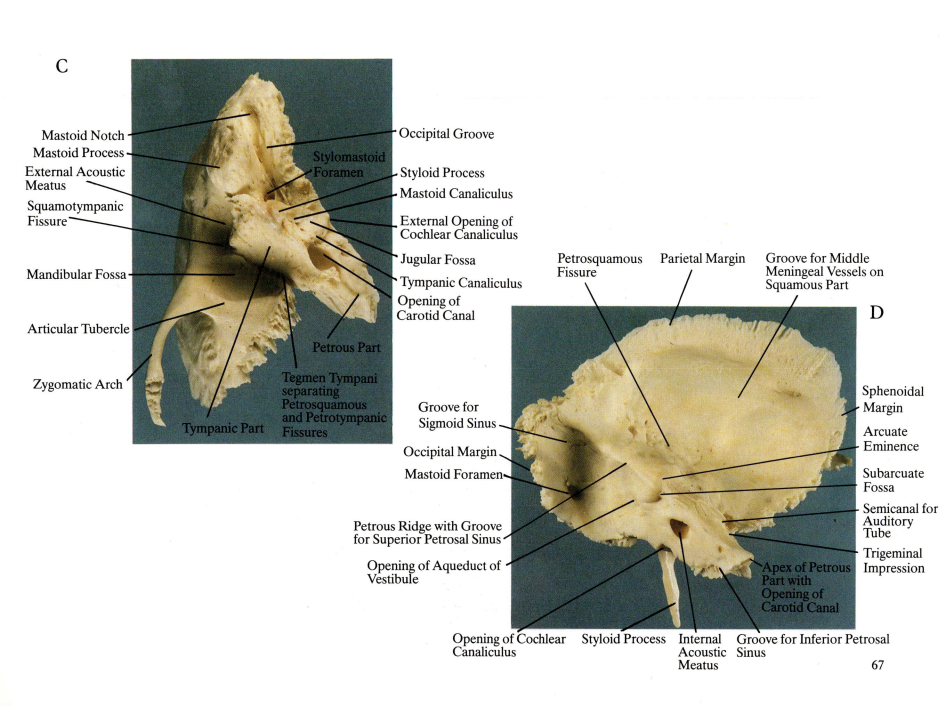

C

Mastoid Notch

Mastoid Process

External Acoustic
Meatus

Squamotympanic
Fissure

Mandibular Fossa

Articular Tubercle

Zygomatic Arch

Tympanic Part

Tegmen Tympani
separating
Petrosquamous
and Petrotympanic
Fissures

Occipital Groove

Stylomastoid
Foramen

Styloid Process

Mastoid Canaliculus

External Opening of
Cochlear Canaliculus

Jugular Fossa

Tympanic Canaliculus

Opening of
Carotid Canal

Petrous Part

D

Petrosquamous
Fissure

Parietal Margin

Groove for Middle
Meningeal Vessels on
Squamous Part

Groove for
Sigmoid Sinus

Occipital Margin

Mastoid Foramen

Petrous Ridge with Groove
for Superior Petrosal Sinus

Opening of Aqueduct of
Vestibule

Sphenoidal
Margin

Arcuate
Eminence

Subarcuate
Fossa

Semicanal for
Auditory
Tube

Trigeminal
Impression

Apex of Petrous
Part with
Opening of
Carotid Canal

Opening of Cochlear
Canaliculus

Styloid Process

Internal
Acoustic
Meatus

Groove for Inferior Petrosal
Sinus

67

SECTION THROUGH TEMPORAL BONE TO SHOW
MEDIAL WALL OF TYMPANIC CAVITY

Site of Geniculate Ganglion
of Facial Nerve

Anterior Semicircular
Canal

Horizontal Part of Facial
Canal

Cochlea

Fenestra Vestibuli

Carotid Canal

Vertical Part of Facial
Canal

Fenestra Cochleae

EAR OSSICLES

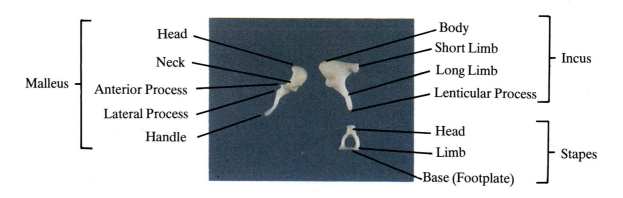

Head

Body

Neck

Short Limb

Anterior Process

Long Limb

Malleus

Lenticular Process

Incus

Lateral Process

Handle

Head

Limb

Stapes

Base (Footplate)

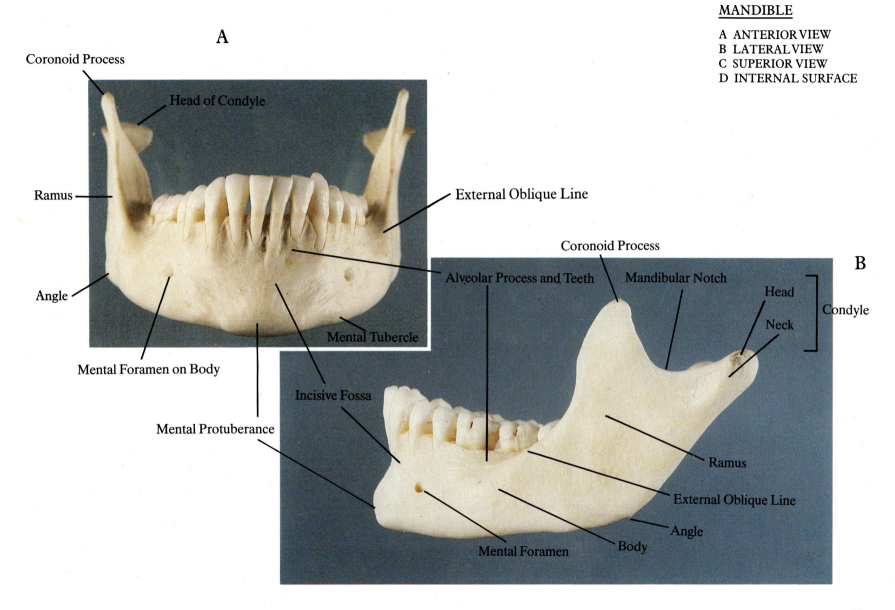

A

Coronoid Process

Head of Condyle

Ramus

Angle

Mental Foramen on Body

Mental Protuberance

External Oblique Line

Alveolar Process and Teeth

Incisive Fossa

Mental Tubercle

B

Coronoid Process

Mandibular Notch

Head

Neck

Condyle

Ramus

External Oblique Line

Angle

Body

Mental Foramen

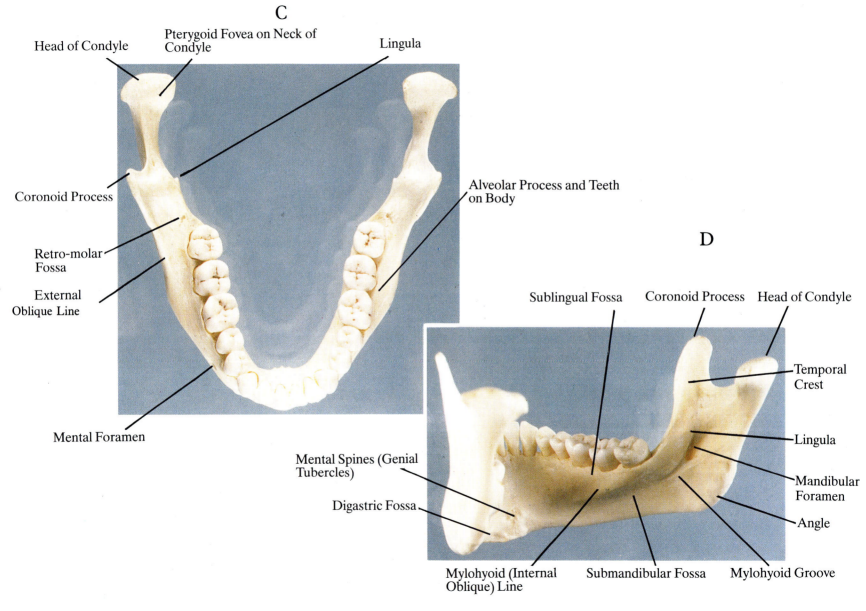

C

Head of Condyle

Pterygoid Fovea on Neck of Condyle

Lingula

Coronoid Process

Retro-molar Fossa

External Oblique Line

Mental Foramen

Alveolar Process and Teeth on Body

D

Sublingual Fossa

Coronoid Process

Head of Condyle

Temporal Crest

Lingula

Mandibular Foramen

Angle

Mylohyoid Groove

Submandibular Fossa

Mylohyoid (Internal Oblique) Line

Mental Spines (Genial Tubercles)

Digastric Fossa

MAXILLARY BONE

A ANTERIOR VIEW
B LATERAL VIEW
C SUPERIOR VIEW
D INFERIOR VIEW
E POSTERIOR VIEW
F MEDIAL VIEW

A

B

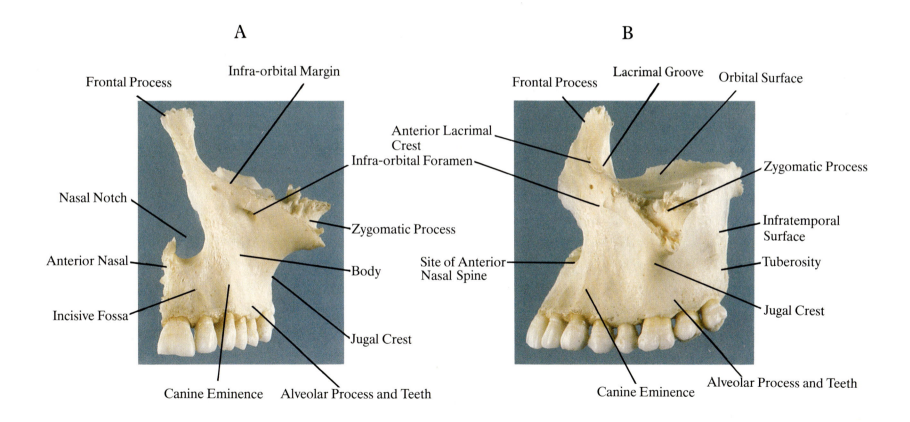

Frontal Process

Infra-orbital Margin

Nasal Notch

Anterior Nasal

Incisive Fossa

Zygomatic Process

Body

Jugal Crest

Canine Eminence   Alveolar Process and Teeth

Frontal Process

Lacrimal Groove   Orbital Surface

Anterior Lacrimal Crest

Infra-orbital Foramen

Site of Anterior Nasal Spine

Zygomatic Process

Infratemporal Surface

Tuberosity

Jugal Crest

Canine Eminence

Alveolar Process and Teeth

C

D

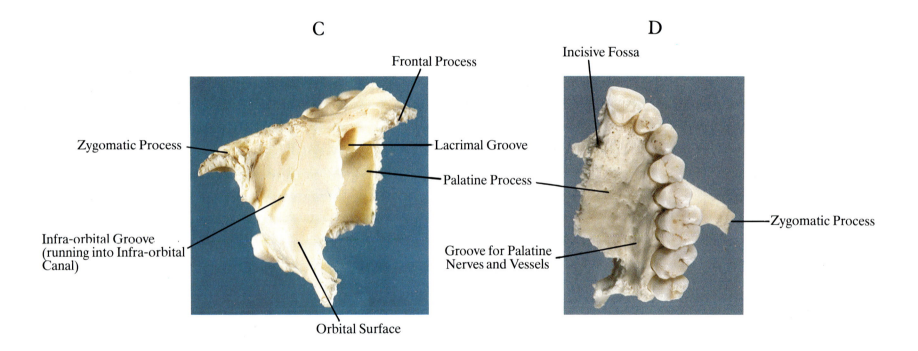

Frontal Process

Zygomatic Process

Infra-orbital Groove
(running into Infra-orbital
Canal)

Orbital Surface

Lacrimal Groove

Palatine Process

Incisive Fossa

Zygomatic Process

Groove for Palatine
Nerves and Vessels

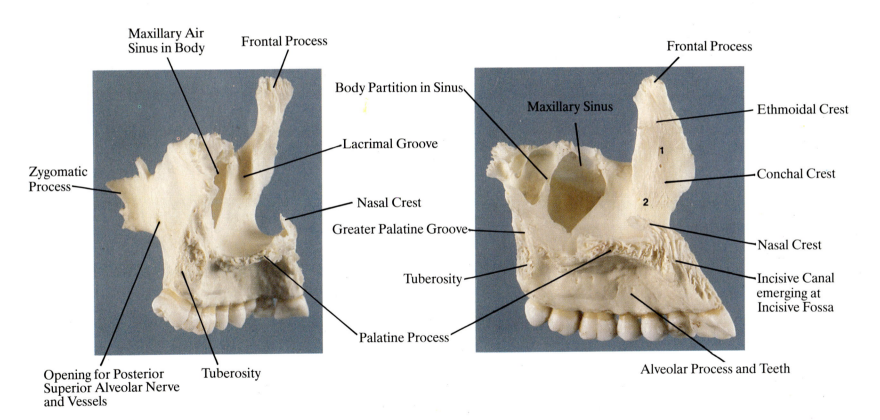

E

Maxillary Air Sinus in Body

Frontal Process

Zygomatic Process

Opening for Posterior Superior Alveolar Nerve and Vessels

Tuberosity

Body Partition in Sinus

Lacrimal Groove

Nasal Crest

Greater Palatine Groove

Tuberosity

Palatine Process

F

Frontal Process

Maxillary Sinus

Ethmoidal Crest

1

Conchal Crest

2

Nasal Crest

Incisive Canal emerging at Incisive Fossa

Alveolar Process and Teeth

1 — Middle Meatus
2 — Inferior Meatus

PALATINE BONE

A ANTERIOR VIEW
B POSTERIOR VIEW
C LATERAL VIEW
D MEDIAL VIEW
E SUPERIOR VIEW
F INFERIOR VIEW

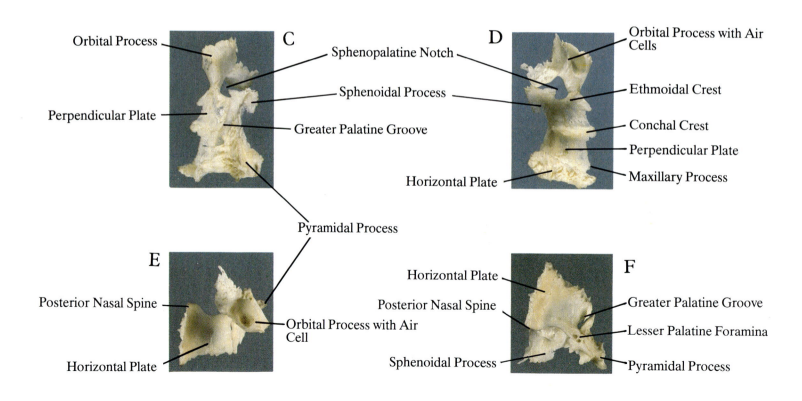

A

Orbital Process with Air Cell

Sphenopalatine Notch

Ethmoidal Crest

Sphenoidal Process

Conchal Crest

Perpendicular Plate

Greater Palatine Groove

Nasal Crest

Pyramidal Process

Horizontal Plate

B

Orbital Process

Sphenoidal Process

Perpendicular Plate

Nasal Crest

Horizontal Plate

C

Orbital Process

Sphenopalatine Notch

Perpendicular Plate

Sphenoidal Process

Greater Palatine Groove

D

Orbital Process with Air Cells

Ethmoidal Crest

Conchal Crest

Perpendicular Plate

Horizontal Plate

Maxillary Process

Pyramidal Process

E

Posterior Nasal Spine

Horizontal Plate

Orbital Process with Air Cell

F

Horizontal Plate

Posterior Nasal Spine

Greater Palatine Groove

Lesser Palatine Foramina

Sphenoidal Process

Pyramidal Process

ZYGOMATIC BONE

A LATERAL VIEW
B MEDIAL VIEW
C ANTERIOR VIEW

A

B

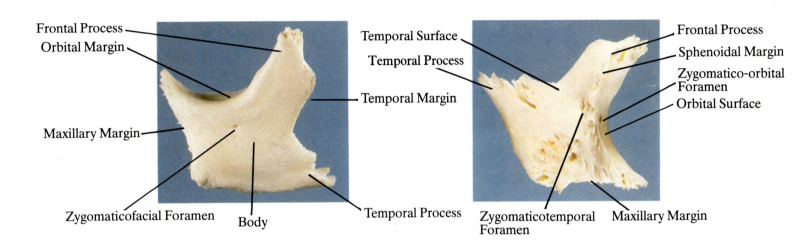

Frontal Process

Orbital Margin

Maxillary Margin

Zygomaticofacial Foramen

Body

Temporal Margin

Temporal Process

Temporal Surface

Temporal Process

Zygomaticotemporal Foramen

Frontal Process

Sphenoidal Margin

Zygomatico-orbital Foramen

Orbital Surface

Maxillary Margin

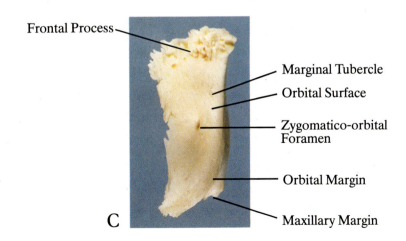

Frontal Process

Marginal Tubercle

Orbital Surface

Zygomatico-orbital Foramen

Orbital Margin

Maxillary Margin

C

INFERIOR NASAL CONCHA

A MEDIAL VIEW
B LATERAL VIEW
C POSTERIOR VIEW

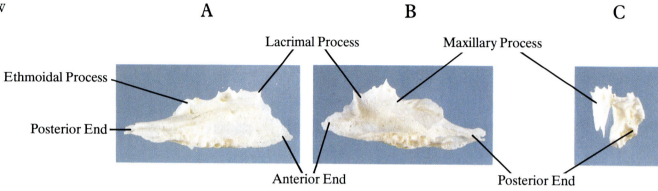

NASAL BONE

A EXTERNAL SURFACE
B INTERNAL SURFACE

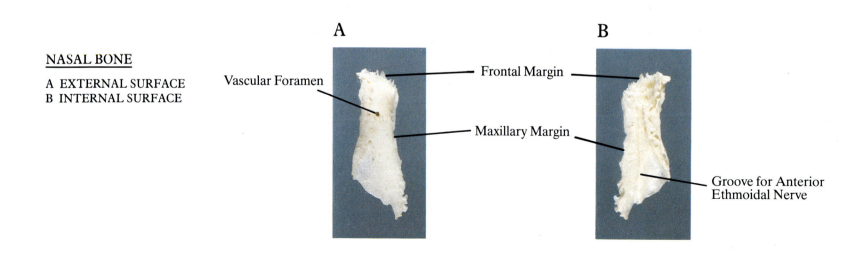

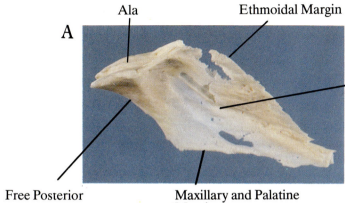

A

Ala

Ethmoidal Margin

Groove for Nasopalatine
Nerve and Vessels

Free Posterior
Border

Maxillary and Palatine
Margin

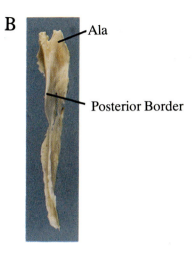

B

Ala

Posterior Border

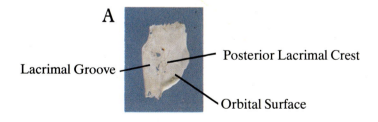

A

Lacrimal Groove

Posterior Lacrimal Crest

Orbital Surface

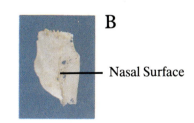

B

Nasal Surface

LACRIMAL BONE

A EXTERNAL SURFACE
B INTERNAL SURFACE

TOOTH
MORPHOLOGY

M an has two generations of teeth, the deciduous (or primary) dentition and the permanent (or secondary) dentition. There are no teeth in the mouth at birth but by the age of three years the deciduous dentition is complete. By six years, the first permanent teeth appear and thence the deciduous teeth are exfoliated one by one to be replaced by their permanent successors. A complete permanent dentition is present at or about 18 years. Thus, given the average life of 70 years, the functional life span of the deciduous dentition is only six per cent of this total, while with care it can be over 90 per cent for the permanent dentition. In the complete deciduous dentition there are 20 teeth—10 in each jaw. In the complete permanent dentition there are 32 teeth—16 in each jaw. In both dentitions, there are three basic tooth forms: incisiform, caniniform and molariform. Incisiform teeth (incisors) are cutting teeth, having thin, blade-like crowns. Caniniform teeth (canines) are piercing or tearing teeth, having a single, stout, pointed, cone-shaped crown. Molariform teeth (molars and premolars) are grinding teeth, possessing a number of cusps on an otherwise flattened biting surface. Premolars are bicuspid teeth which are particular to the permanent dentition and which replace the deciduous molars.

The types and numbers of teeth can be expressed using dental formulae. The type of tooth is represented by its initial letter (i.e. I for incisors, C for canines, P for premolars and M for molars). The deciduous dentition is indicated by the letter D. The formula for the deciduous dentition of man is $DI^2/_2DC^1/_1DM^2/_2 = 10$, and for the permanent dentition $I^2/_2C^1/_1P^2/_2M^3/_3 = 16$, where the numbers following each letter refer to the number of teeth of each type in the upper and lower jaws on one side only.

Identification of teeth is made not only according to the dentition to which they belong and to basic tooth form, but also according to their anatomical location within the jaws. The tooth-bearing region of the jaws can be divided into four quadrants, the right and left maxillary and mandibular quadrants. A tooth may thus be identified according to the quadrant in which it is located, e.g. a right maxillary deciduous incisor or a left mandibular permanent molar. In both the permanent and deciduous dentitions, the incisors may be distinguished according to their relationship to the midline. Thus, the incisor nearest the midline is the central or first incisor, the incisor which is more laterally positioned being termed the lateral or second incisor. The permanent premolars and the permanent and deciduous molars can also be distinguished according to their mesiodistal relationships. The molar most mesially positioned is designated the first molar, the one behind it being the second molar. In the permanent dentition, the tooth most distally positioned is the third molar. The mesial premolar is the first premolar, the premolar behind it being the second premolar.

A dental shorthand may be used in the clinic to simplify tooth identification. The permanent teeth in each quadrant are numbered 1 to 8 and the deciduous teeth in each quadrant are lettered A to E.

The symbols for the quadrants are derived from an imaginary cross with the horizontal bar placed between the upper and lower jaw and the vertical bar running between the upper and lower central incisors.

UPPER RIGHT =| |= UPPER LEFT

LOWER RIGHT =| |= LOWER LEFT

Thus, the maxillary right first permanent molar is allocated the symbol 6| and the mandibular left deciduous canine |C. This system of dental shorthand is termed the Zsigmondy System. An alternative scheme has been devised by the Federation Dentaire Internationale in which the quadrant is represented by a number

1 = maxillary right quadrant	
2 = maxillary left quadrant	
3 = mandibular left quadrant	Permanent
4 = mandibular right quadrant	
5 = maxillary right quadrant	
6 = maxillary left quadrant	
7 = mandibular left quadrant	Deciduous
8 = mandibular right quadrant	

which prefixes a tooth number. According to this system, the maxillary right first permanent molar is symbolised as 1,6 and the mandibular left deciduous canine as 7,3.

Some terms used for the description of tooth form:

Crown   Clinical crown—that portion of a tooth visible in the oral cavity.
Anatomical crown—that portion of a tooth covered with enamel.

Root   Clinical root—that portion of a tooth which lies within the alveolus.
Anatomical root—that portion of a tooth covered by cementum.

Cervical margin   The junction of the anatomical crown and root.

Occlusal surface   The biting surface of a molar or premolar.

Incisal margin   The cutting edge of incisor teeth, analogous to the occlusal surface of the molariform teeth.

Cusp   A pronounced elevation on the occlusal surface of a tooth.

Tubercle   A small elevation on the crown which may or may not be typical.

Cingulum   A bulbous convexity near the cervical region of a tooth.

Ridge   A linear elevation on the surface of a tooth.

Marginal ridge   A ridge at the mesial or distal edge of the occlusal surface of molariform teeth. Maxillary incisors and canine teeth may have equivalent ridges.

Fissure   A long cleft between cusps or ridges.

Fossa   A rounded depression in the surface of a tooth.

Buccal   Towards or adjacent to the cheek. The term buccal surface is reserved for that surface of a premolar or molar which is positioned immediately adjacent to the cheek.

Labial   Towards or adjacent to the lips. The term labial surface is reserved for that surface of an incisor or canine which is positioned immediately adjacent to the lips.

Palatal   Towards or adjacent to the palate. The term palatal surface is reserved for that surface of a maxillary tooth which is positioned immediately adjacent to the palate.

Lingual   Towards or adjacent to the tongue. The term lingual surface is reserved for that surface of a mandibular tooth which lies immediately adjacent to the tongue.

Mesial   Towards the median. The mesial surface is that surface which faces towards the median line following the curve of the dental arch.

Distal   Away from the median. The distal surface is that surface which faces away from the median line following the curve of the dental arch.

THE MORPHOLOGY OF THE PERMANENT TEETH

The Incisors

The incisors of man have thin, blade-like crowns which are adapted for the cutting and shearing of food preparatory to grinding. They have single roots. Viewed mesially or distally, the crowns of the incisors are roughly triangular in shape, with the apex of the triangle at the incisal margin of the tooth. This shape is thought to facilitate the penetration and cutting of food. Viewed buccally or lingually, the incisors are trapezoidal, the shortest of the uneven sides being the base of the crown cervically.

The mandibular incisors have the smallest mesiodistal dimensions of any teeth in the permanent dentition. They can be distinguished from the maxillary incisors not only by their size but also by the marked lingual inclination of the crowns over the roots, the mesiodistal compression of their roots and the poor development of the marginal ridges and cingula.

The Canines

Canines are the only teeth in the dentition with a single cusp. Morphologically, they can be considered transitional between incisors and premolars. They have single prominent roots. The mandibular canine can be distinguished from the maxillary tooth as it appears more slender and more symmetrical. Its cusp is generally less-well developed.

The Premolars

Premolars are unique to the permanent dentition. They are sometimes referred to as 'bicuspids', having two main cusps—a buccal and a palatal (or lingual) cusp—which are separated by a mesiodistal occlusal fissure. Premolars are considered to be transitional between canines and molars. The premolar teeth have single roots, except for the maxillary first premolar which has two.

A mandibular premolar differs from a maxillary premolar in that the crown appears rounder when viewed occlusally and the cusps are of unequal size, the buccal cusp being the most prominent. Furthermore, unlike the maxillary premolars, the first and second premolars differ more markedly.

The Molars

Molars present the largest occlusal surfaces of all teeth. They have three to five major cusps. Molars are the only teeth which have more than one buccal cusp. Generally, the lower molars have two roots, the upper, three. The permanent molars do not have deciduous predecessors. Like the premolars, the maxillary molars are roughly trapezoidal when viewed mesially and distally whereas the mandibular molars are rhomboidal. Viewed buccally or lingually, the molars are trapezoidal.

The mandibular molars differ from the maxillary molars in the following respects:

1 the mandibular molars have two roots (one mesial and one distal);
2 they are considered to be derived from a five-cusped form;
3 the crowns of the mandibular molars are oblong, being broader mesiodistally than buccolingually;
4 the fissure pattern is cross-shaped;
5 the lingual cusps are of more equal size;
6 the tips of the buccal cusps are shifted lingually so that from the occlusal view the whole of the buccal surface is visible.

THE MORPHOLOGY OF THE DECIDUOUS TEETH

The morphology of the deciduous incisors and canines resembles that of their respective permanent successors. The second deciduous molars are similar to the adjacent first permanent molars. Thus, only the first deciduous molars have distinct morphologies. The first maxillary deciduous molar is intermediate in form between a premolar and a molar. Viewed occlusally, the crown is an irregular quadrilateral, the mesiopalatal angle being markedly obtuse. It is generally bicuspid and has three divergent roots. A prominent bulge (the molar tubercle) lies at the mesiobuccal corner of the crown, near the mesiobuccal root. The first mandibular molar is molariform. Viewed occlusally, the crown appears elongated mesiodistally and the mesiolingual angle is markedly obtuse. Four low cusps are present, the mesiobuccal cusp being the largest. A bulge (the molar tubercle) lies at the mesiobuccal corner of the crown. Two divergent roots are present, mesial and distal.

For a full written description of the permanent and deciduous dentition, the reader is referred to:
A Colour Atlas and Textbook of Oral Anatomy by B.K.B. Berkovitz, G.R. Holland, and B.J. Moxham (Wolfe Publishing, 1978).

Principal differences between the permanent and deciduous dentitions

1 The dental formula for the deciduous dentition is:
$$DI^2/_2DC^1/_1DM^2/_2 = 10$$
while that of the permanent dentition is:
$$I^2/_2C^1/_1P^2/_2M^3/_3 = 16.$$

2 The deciduous teeth are smaller than their corresponding permanent successors though the mesiodistal dimensions of the permanent premolars are generally less than those for the deciduous molars.

3 Deciduous teeth have a greater constancy of shape.

4 The crowns of deciduous teeth appear bulbous, often having pronounced labial or buccal cingula.

5 The cervical margins of deciduous teeth are more sharply demarcated and pronounced than those of the permanent teeth, the enamel bulging at the cervical margins rather than gently tapering.

6 Comparing newly-erupted teeth, the cusps of deciduous teeth are more pointed than those of the permanent teeth.

7 The crowns of deciduous teeth have a thinner covering of enamel (average width 0.5mm-1.0mm) than the crowns of permanent teeth (average width 2.5mm).

8 The enamel of deciduous teeth, being more opaque than that of permanent teeth, gives the crown a whiter appearance.

9 The enamel of deciduous teeth is softer than that of permanent teeth and is more easily worn.

10 The enamel of deciduous teeth is more permeable than that of permanent teeth.

11 The roots of deciduous teeth are shorter and less robust than those of the permanent teeth.

12 The roots of the deciduous incisors and canines are longer in proportion to the crown than those of their permanent counterparts.

13 The roots of the deciduous molars are widely divergent, extending beyond the dimensions of the crown.

14 The pulp chambers of deciduous teeth are proportionally larger in relation to the crown than those of the permanent teeth. The pulp horns in deciduous teeth are more prominent.

15 The root canals of deciduous teeth are extremely fine.

The pictures of the teeth in this atlas are enlarged by $\times 1^1/_2$. The permanent teeth are described before the deciduous teeth, and within each dentition the maxillary teeth are presented before the mandibular teeth. The maxillary and mandibular third permanent molars are not illustrated because of the great variation in their morphology. In all instances, the teeth shown are from the left side of the dentition. To help visualise the tooth as a three dimensional object, the illustrations of each tooth are arranged according to the 'third angle projection technique' which aligns each side of a tooth around a central view of its occlusal or incisal aspect.

In the illustrations B = buccal surface, D = distal surface, L = lingual surface, La = labial surface, M = mesial surface, P = palatal surface, O = occlusal, or incisal, surface.

OCCLUSAL VIEWS OF THE DENTITION

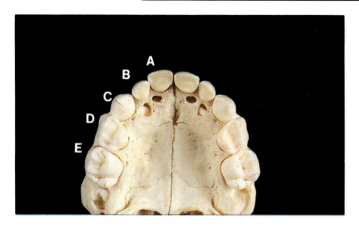

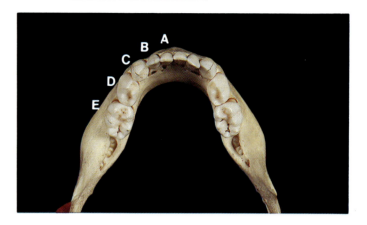

COMPLETE DECIDUOUS DENTITION

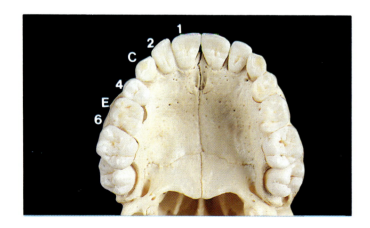

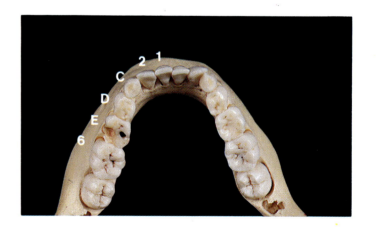

MIXED DENTITION

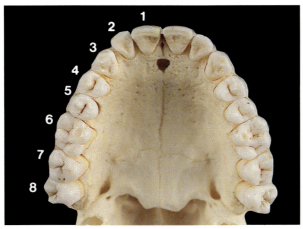

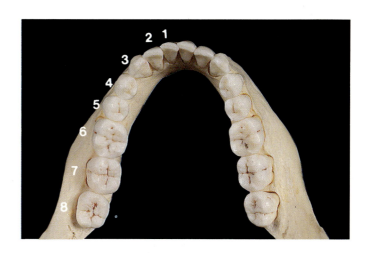

COMPLETE PERMANENT DENTITION

THE PERMANENT DENTITION

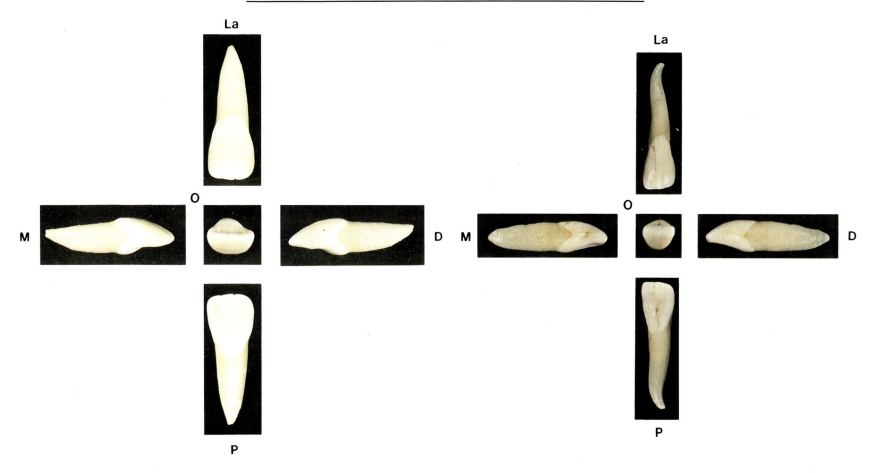

La

O

M

D

P

La

O

M

D

P

MAXILLARY FIRST (CENTRAL) INCISOR (⌐1; 2,1)

MAXILLARY SECOND (LATERAL) INCISOR (⌐2; 2,2)

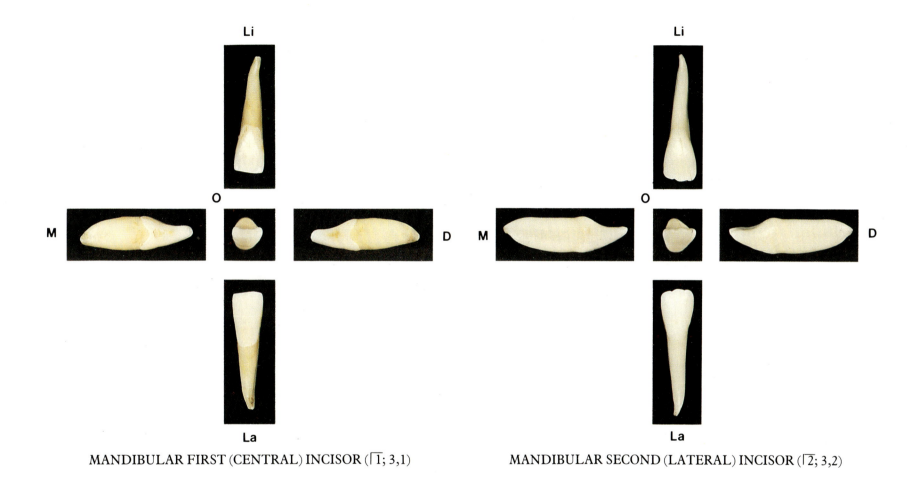

Li

O

M   D

La

MANDIBULAR FIRST (CENTRAL) INCISOR ($\overline{1}$; 3,1)

Li

O

M   D

La

MANDIBULAR SECOND (LATERAL) INCISOR ($\overline{2}$; 3,2)

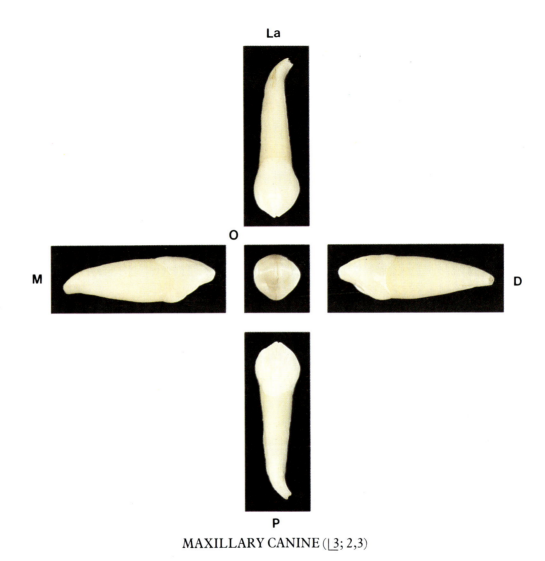

La

O

M

D

P

MAXILLARY CANINE (⌊3; 2,3)

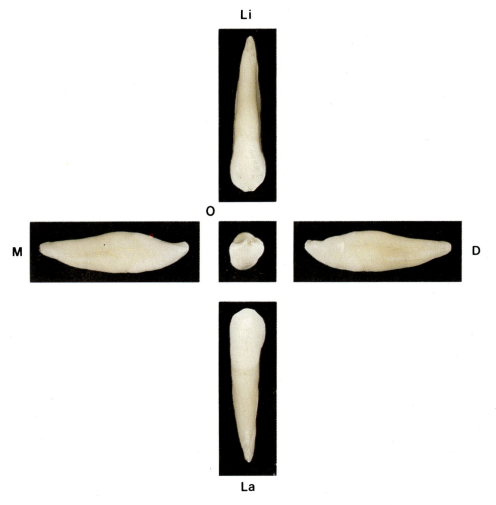

MANDIBULAR CANINE ($\overline{3}$; 3,3)

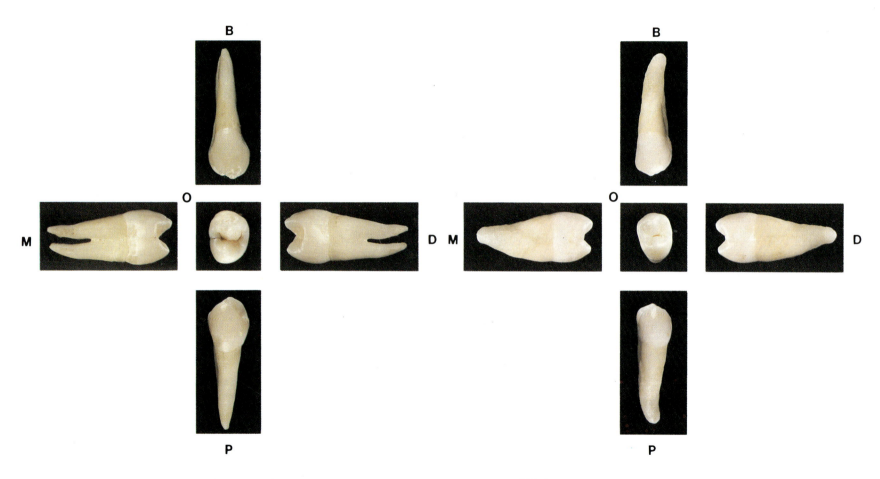

B

O

M

D

P

MAXILLARY FIRST PREMOLAR (⌊4; 2,4)

B

O

M

D

P

MAXILLARY SECOND PREMOLAR (⌊5; 2,5)

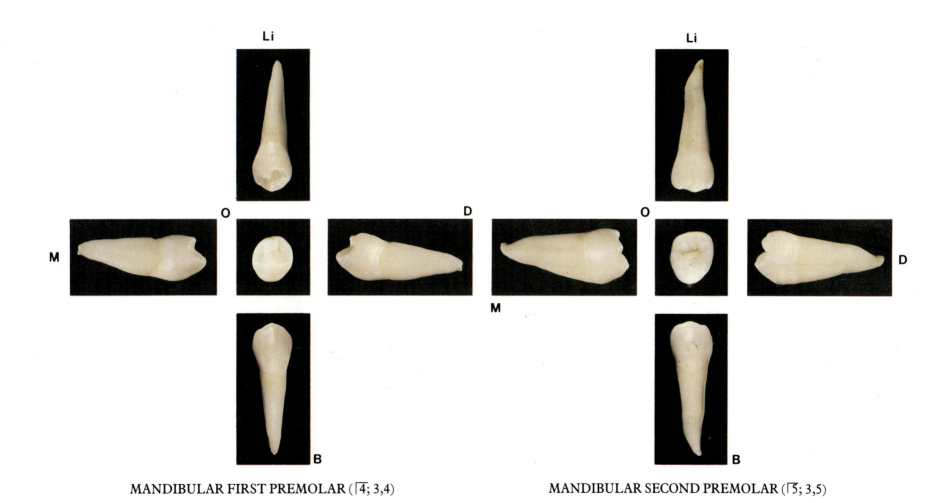

Li

O

M

D

B

MANDIBULAR FIRST PREMOLAR ($\overline{4}$; 3,4)

Li

O

M

D

B

MANDIBULAR SECOND PREMOLAR ($\overline{5}$; 3,5)

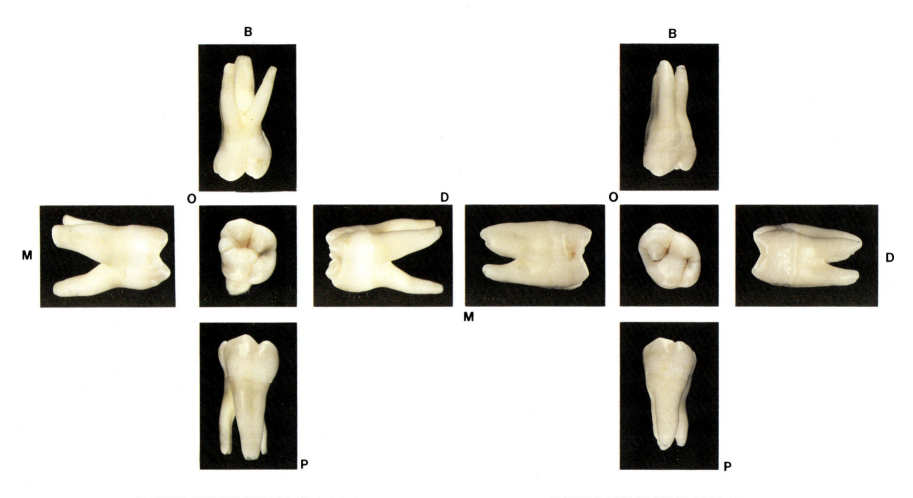

MAXILLARY FIRST MOLAR (|6; 2,6)   MAXILLARY SECOND MOLAR (|7; 2,7)

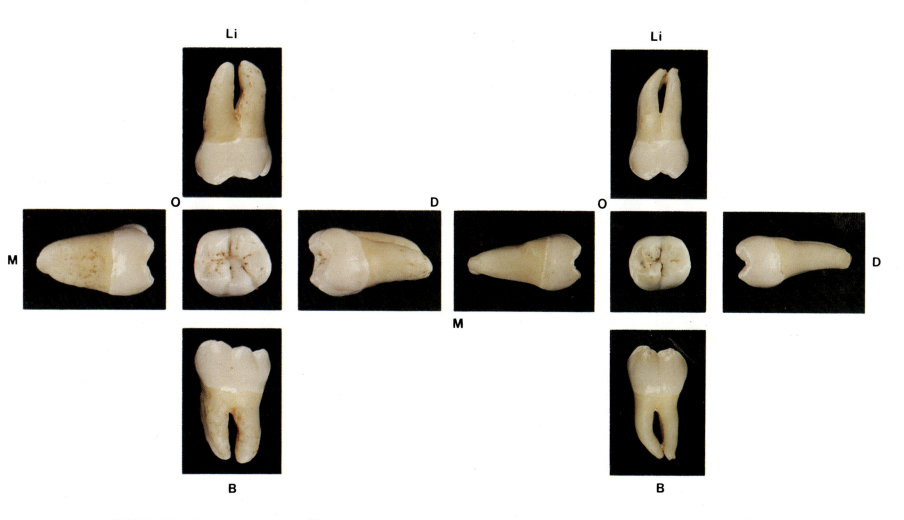

Li

O

D

M

M

B

D

Li

O

M

B

MANDIBULAR FIRST MOLAR ($\overline{6}$; 3,6)

MANDIBULAR SECOND MOLAR ($\overline{7}$; 3,7)

THE DECIDUOUS DENTITION

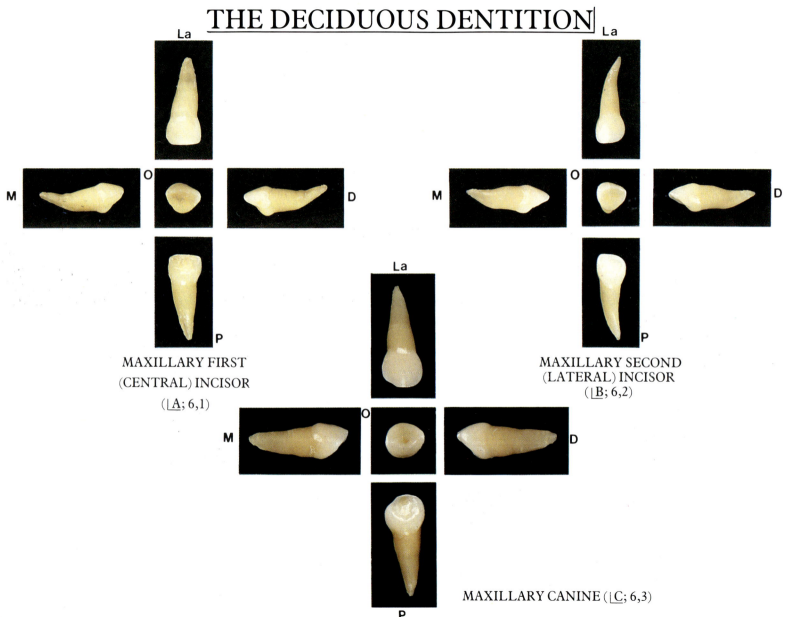

MAXILLARY FIRST
(CENTRAL) INCISOR
(⌞A; 6,1)

MAXILLARY SECOND
(LATERAL) INCISOR
(⌞B; 6,2)

MAXILLARY CANINE (⌞C; 6,3)

MANDIBULAR FIRST
(CENTRAL) INCISOR
($\overline{A}$; 7,1)

MANDIBULAR SECOND
(LATERAL) INCISOR
($\overline{B}$; 7,2)

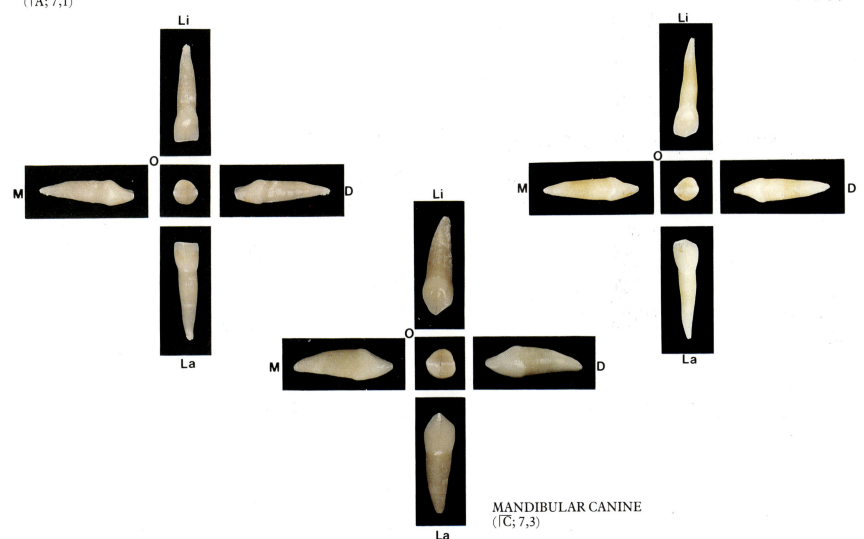

Li

M   O   D

La

Li

M   O   D

La

Li

M   O   D

La

MANDIBULAR CANINE
($\overline{C}$; 7,3)

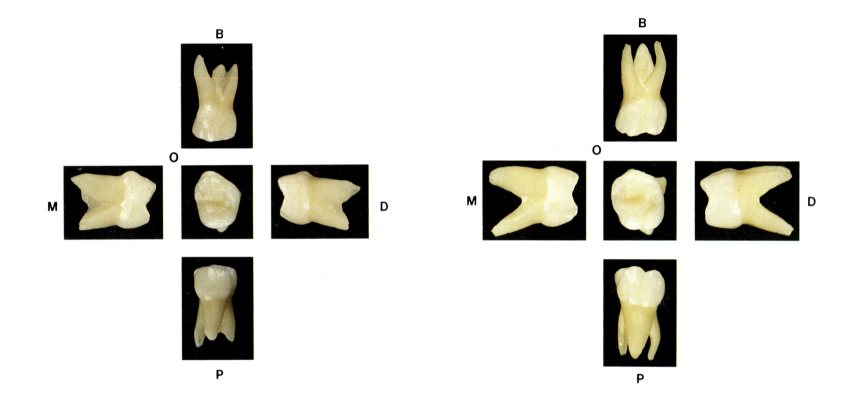

B

O

M

D

P

MAXILLARY FIRST MOLAR (⌊D; 6,4)

B

O

M

D

P

MAXILLARY SECOND MOLAR (⌊E; 6,5)

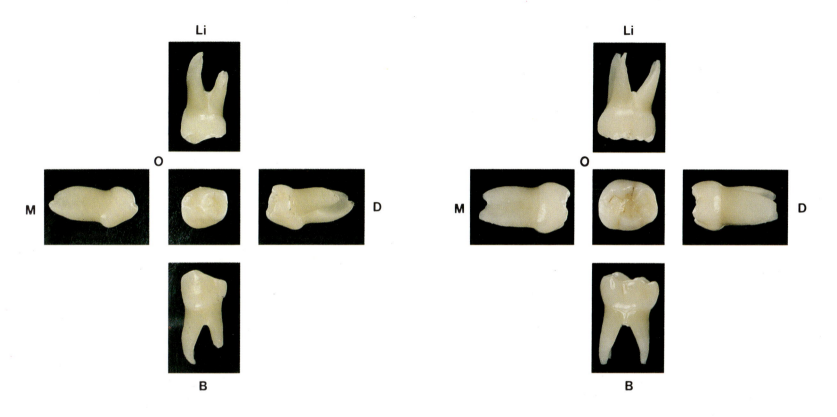

Li

O

M   D

B

Li

O

M   D

B

MANDIBULAR FIRST MOLAR ($\overline{\text{D}}$; 7,4)

MANDIBULAR SECOND MOLAR ($\overline{\text{E}}$; 7,5)

CHRONOLOGY OF TOOTH DEVELOPMENT

CHRONOLOGY OF THE DECIDUOUS DENTITION

Tooth	First evidence of calcification (months I.U.)	Crown completed (months)	Eruption (months)	Root completed (years)
Maxillary				
A	3-4	4	7	1½-2
B	4½	5	8	1½-2
C	5	9	16-20	2½-3
D	5	6	12-16	2-2½
E	6-7	10-12	21-30	3
Mandibular				
A	4½	4	6½	1½-2
B	4½	4½	7	1½-2
C	5	9	16-20	2½-3
D	5	6	12-16	2-2½
E	6	10-12	21-30	3

Unless otherwise indicated all dates are post-partum. I.U. = *In utero*. The teeth are identified according to the Zsigmondy System.

CHRONOLOGY OF THE PERMANENT DENTITION

Tooth	First evidence of calcification	Crown completed (years)	Eruption (years)	Root completed (years)
Maxillary				
1	3-4 months	4-5	7-8	10
2	10-12 months	4-5	8-9	11
3	4-5 months	6-7	11-12	13-15
4	1½-1¾ years	5-6	10-11	12-13
5	2-2½ years	6-7	10-12	12-14
6	Birth	2½-3	6-7	9-10
7	2½-3 years	7-8	12-13	14-16
8	7-9 years	12-16	17-21	18-25
Mandibular				
1	3-4 months	4-5	6-7	9
2	3-4 months	4-5	7-8	10
3	4-5 months	6-7	9-10	12-14
4	1¾-2 years	5-6	10-12	12-13
5	2¼-2½ years	6-7	11-12	13-14
6	Birth	2½-3	6-7	9-10
7	2½-3 years	7-8	12-13	14-15
8	8-10 years	12-16	17-21	18-25

All dates are post-partum. Teeth are identified according to the Zsigmondy System.

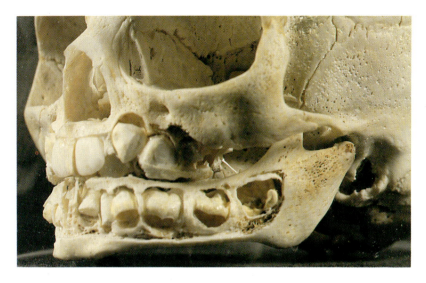

DENTITION AT 4 MONTHS

TEETH ERUPTED   —

TEETH UNERUPTED MAX. <u>A B C D E 6</u>
          MAND. A B C D E 6

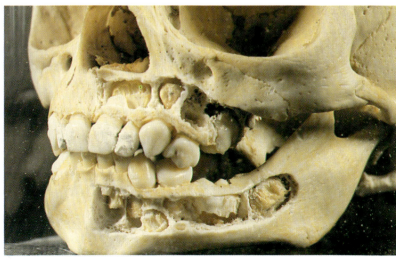

DENTITION AT 1½ YEARS

TEETH ERUPTED   MAX. <u>A B C D</u>
        MAND. A B C D

TEETH UNERUPTED MAX. <u>1 2 3 E 6</u>
          MAND. 1 2 3 E 6

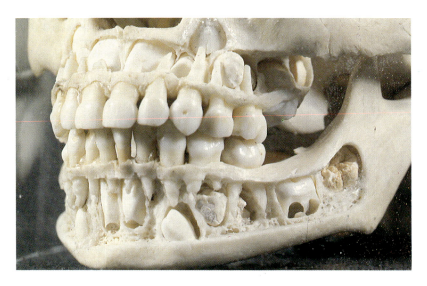

DENTITION AT 4 YEARS

TEETH ERUPTED
MAX. A B C D E
MAND. A B C D E

TEETH UNERUPTED
MAX. 1 2 3 4 5 6 7
MAND. 1 2 3 4 5 6 7

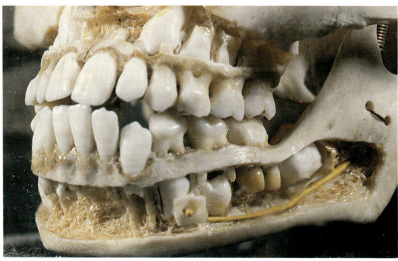

DENTITION AT 9 YEARS

TEETH ERUPTED
MAX. 1 2 C D E 6
MAND. 1 2 3 D E 6

TEETH UNERUPTED
MAX. 7 4 5
MAND. 7 4 5

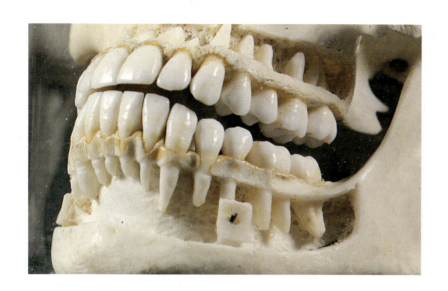

DENTITION AT 15 YEARS

TEETH ERUPTED

MAX. <u>1 2 3 4 5 6 7</u>

MAND. 1 2 3 4 5 6 7

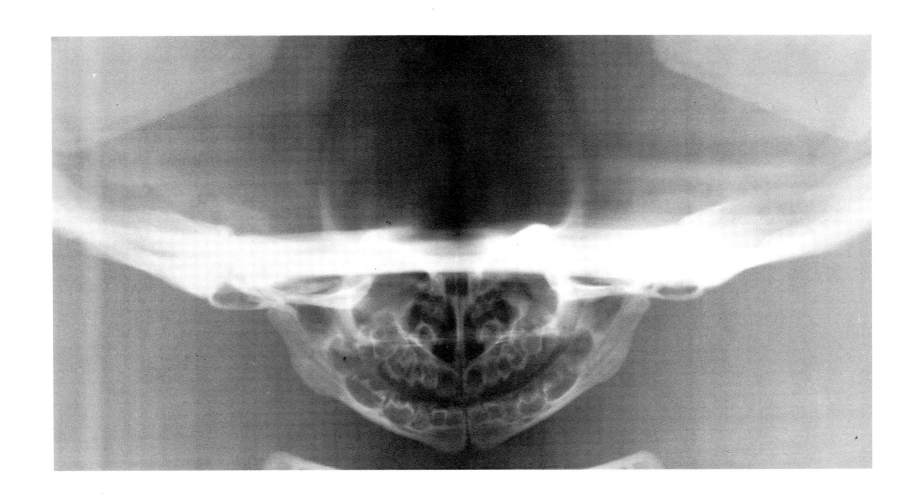

ORTHOPANTOMOGRAM OF DENTITION OF NEONATE

TEETH ERUPTED   —

TEETH UNERUPTED   MAX.   A B C D E 6
                          MAND. A B C D E 6

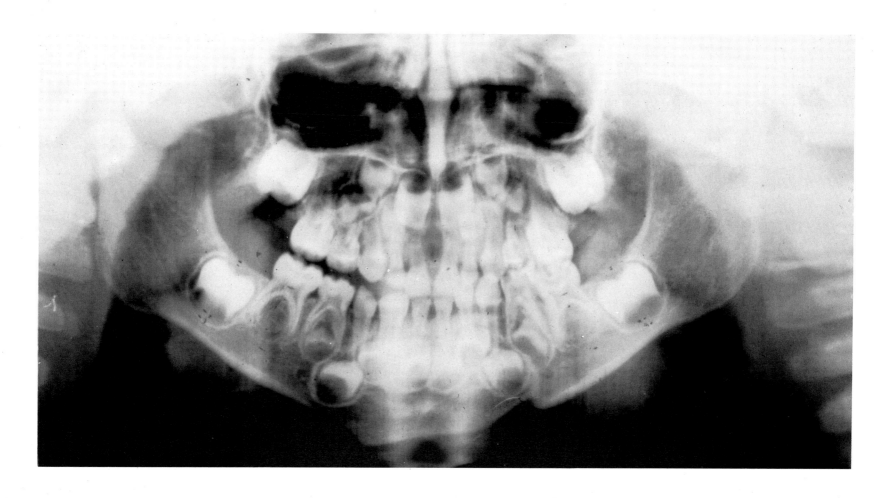

ORTHOPANTOMOGRAM OF DENTITION AT 2½ YEARS

| TEETH ERUPTED | MAX. | <u>A B C D E</u> |
| | MAND. | A B C D E |

| TEETH UNERUPTED | MAX. | <u>1 2 3 4 5 6</u> |
| | MAND. | 1 2 3 4 5 6 |

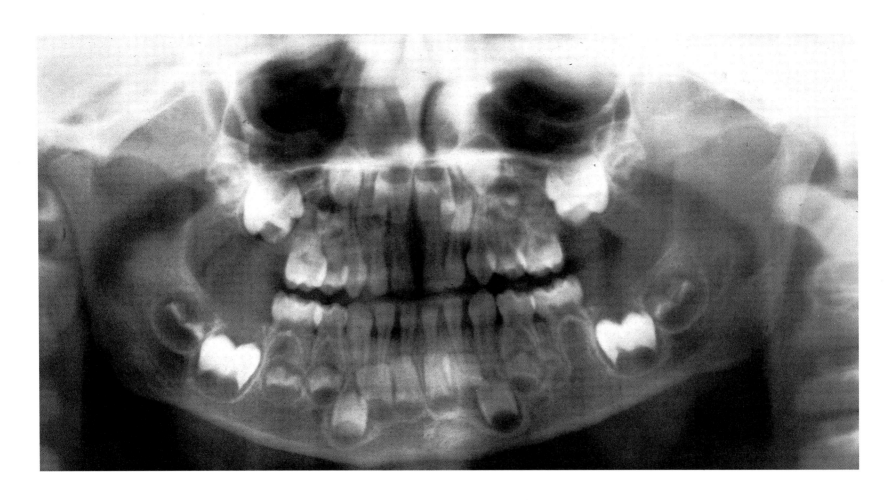

ORTHOPANTOMOGRAM OF DENTITION AT 4 YEARS

TEETH ERUPTED	MAX.	A B C D E
	MAND.	A B C D E
TEETH UNERUPTED	MAX.	1 2 3 4 5 6 7
	MAND.	1 2 3 4 5 6 7

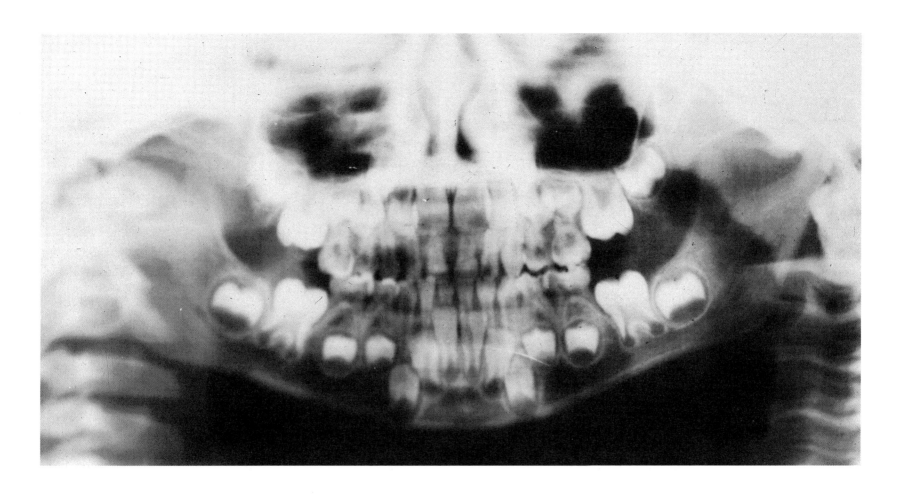

ORTHOPANTOMOGRAM OF DENTITION AT 5½ YEARS

| TEETH ERUPTED | MAX. | A B C D E |
| | MAND. | A B C D E |

| TEETH UNERUPTED | MAX. | 1 2 3 4 5 6 7 |
| | MAND. | 1 2 3 4 5 6 7 |

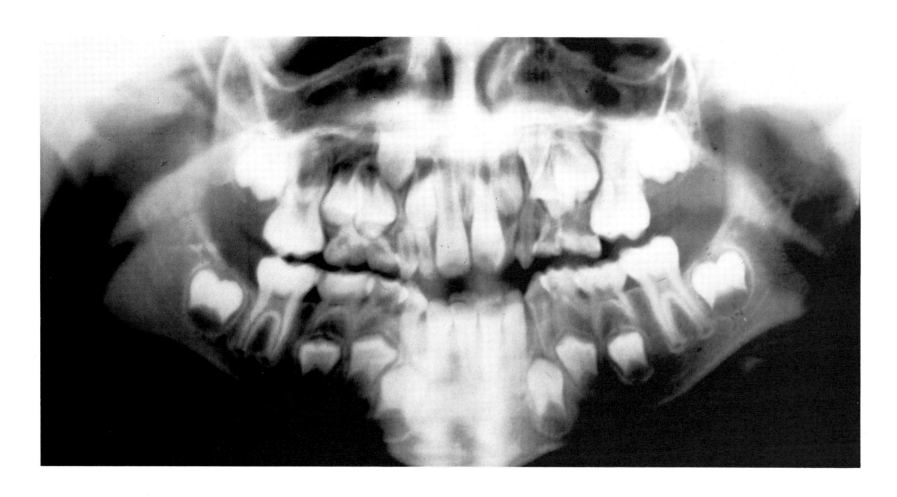

ORTHOPANTOMOGRAM OF DENTITION AT 7 YEARS

| TEETH ERUPTED | MAX. | 1 B C D E 6 |
| | MAND. | 1 2 C D E 6 |

| TEETH UNERUPTED | MAX. | 2 3 4 5 7 |
| | MAND. | 3 4 5 7 |

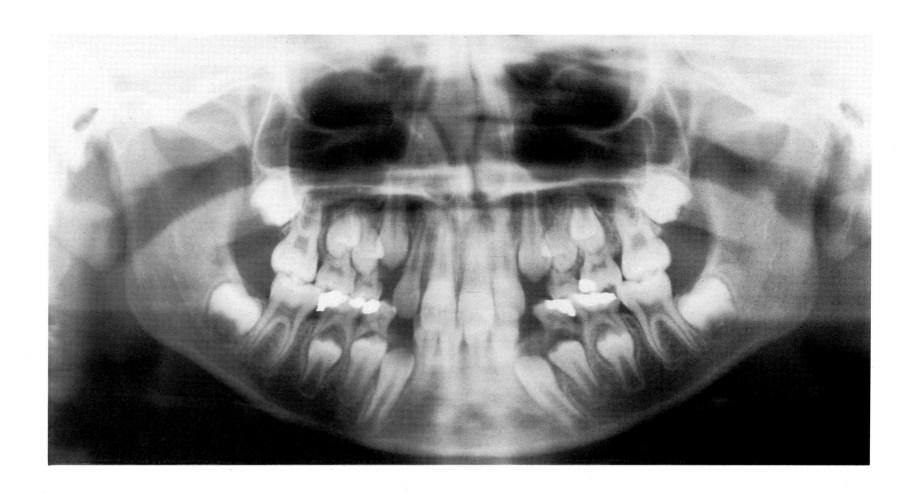

ORTHOPANTOMOGRAM OF DENTITION AT 9 YEARS

TEETH ERUPTED	MAX.	1 2 D E 6
	MAND.	1 2 D E 6

TEETH UNERUPTED	MAX.	3 4 5 7
	MAND.	3 4 5 7

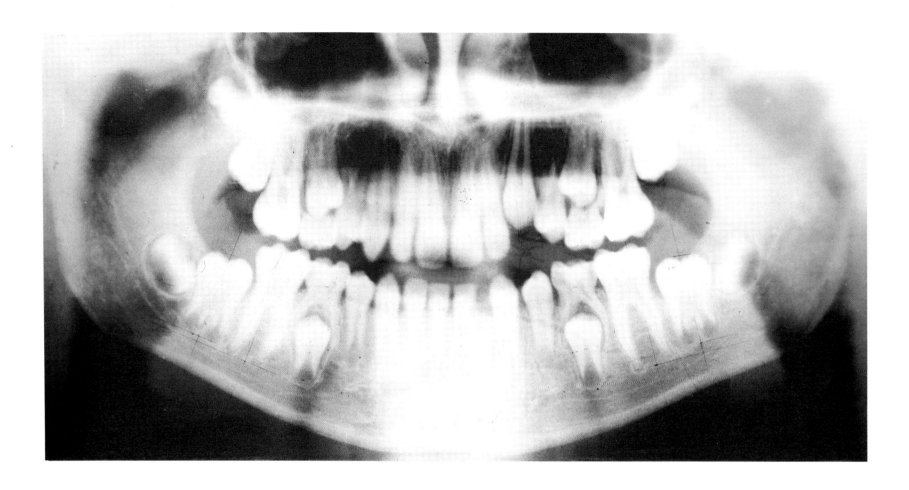

ORTHOPANTOMOGRAM OF DENTITION AT 11 YEARS

| TEETH ERUPTED | MAX. | 1 2 3 4 E 6 |
| | MAND. | 1 2 3 4 E 6 |

| TEETH UNERUPTED | MAX. | 5 7 8 |
| | MAND. | 5 7 8 |

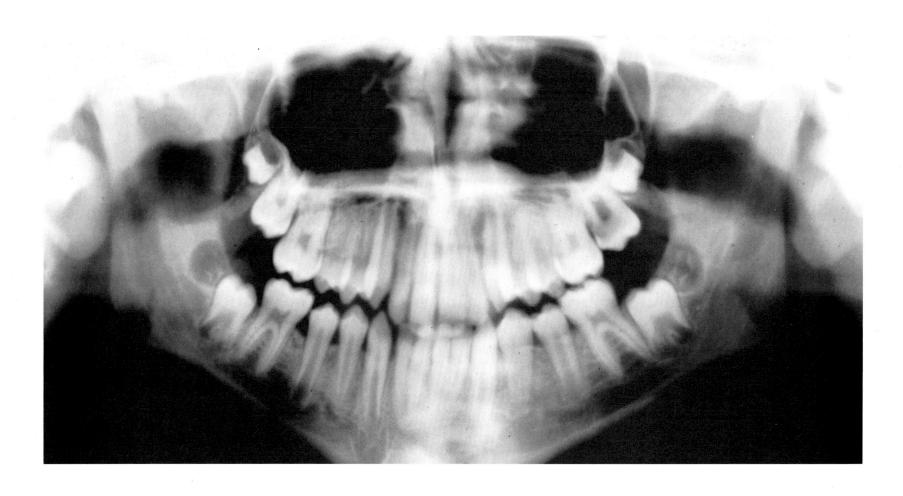

ORTHOPANTOMOGRAM OF DENTITION AT 12 YEARS

TEETH ERUPTED	MAX.	1 2 3 4 5 6
	MAND.	1 2 3 4 5 6

TEETH UNERUPTED	MAX.	7 8
	MAND.	7 8

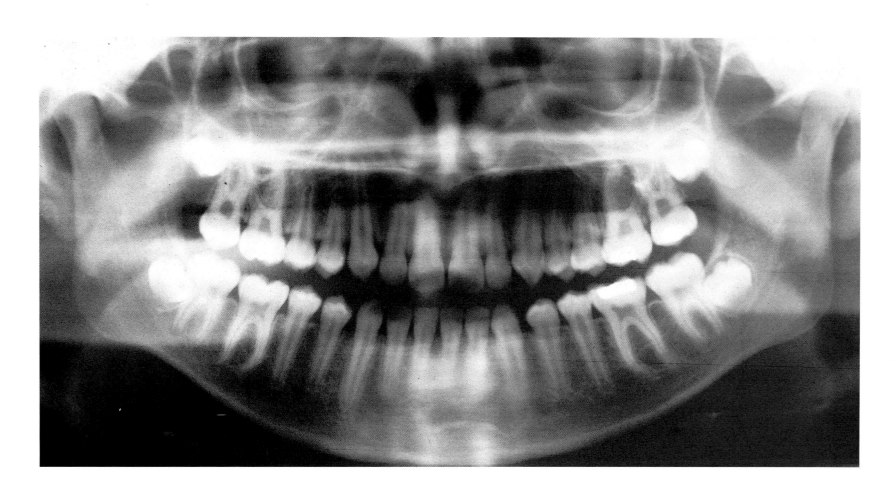

ORTHOPANTOMOGRAM OF DENTITION AT 14 YEARS

TEETH ERUPTED	MAX.	<u>1 2 3 4 5 6 7</u>
	MAND.	1 2 3 4 5 6 7
TEETH UNERUPTED	MAX.	<u>8</u>
	MAND.	8

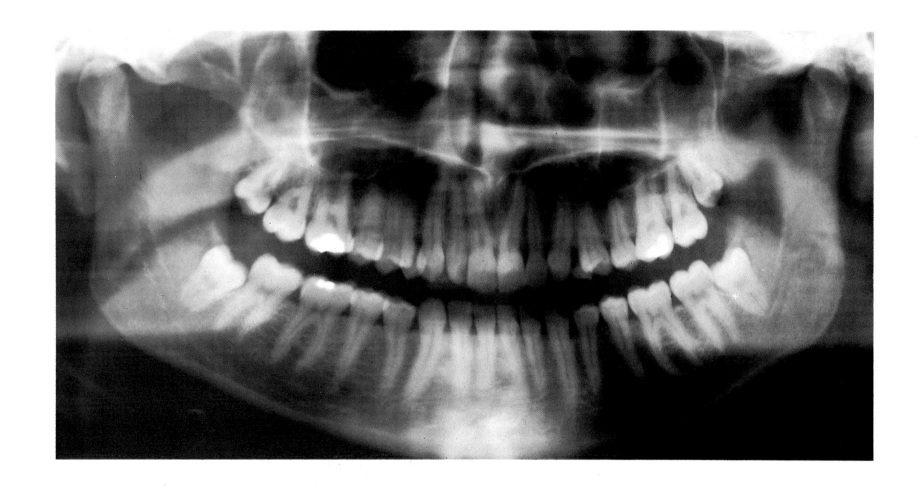

ORTHOPANTOMOGRAM OF DENTITION AT 23 YEARS

TEETH ERUPTED	MAX.	<u>1 2 3 4 5 6 7 8</u>
	MAND.	1 2 3 4 5 6 7 8

INDEX

*Page numbers in **bold** indicate illustrations*